THE PSYCHOLOGICAL CONTEXT OF LABOUR PAIN

PAIN AND ITS ORIGINS, DIAGNOSIS AND TREATMENTS

Additional books in this series can be found on Nova's website under the Series tab.

Additional e-books in this series can be found on Nova's website under the e-book tab.

OBSTETRICS AND GYNECOLOGY ADVANCES

Additional books in this series can be found on Nova's website under the Series tab.

Additional e-books in this series can be found on Nova's website under the e-book tab.

THE PSYCHOLOGICAL CONTEXT OF LABOUR PAIN

JAROSLAVA RAUDENSKÁ
AND
ALENA JAVŮRKOVÁ
EDITORS

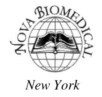

New York

NOTICE TO THE READER

Library of Congress Cataloging-in-Publication Data

ISBN: 978-1-63483-825-2
Library of Congress Control Number: 2015958291

Published by Nova Science Publishers, Inc. † New York

We would like to dedicate this book to our beloved children,
Filip and Ema

CONTENTS

PREFACE

The aim of this book is to explore the relationship between the value and meaning of labour pain and the related psychological, social and cultural context in which it occurs. Filling a gap in the existing literature, we wanted to provide healthcare professionals with an opportunity to reflect upon the topic. In writing our book we also had in mind those primarily concerned with the topic: pregnant women and women in labour, their partners, families and the entire society. A woman's right to choose, among other things, the method of birth and the methods of relieving pain during labour and birth has recently become the topic of heated discussion; this book is our contribution to encourage not only professional, but a wider public debate. The book has six chapters. In selecting the theme of each chapter, we focused on what we perceive as topical issues: the impact of natural childbirth and prophylaxis on the current situation in obstetrics; psychological and social aspects of labour pain; coping strategies; the fear of labour pain and the treatment of fear; a woman's desire for Caesarean section "on demand" and the fear of labour and birth.

Chapter One covers the subject of coping with labour pain and the related social and cultural context, with a particular emphasis on the second half of 20th century. This period witnessed significant changes in the psychological understanding of labour pain and introduced new concepts: natural childbirth and psychoprophylaxis. The chapter focuses on the relationship between healthcare professionals and female patients and the impact of such a relationship on the meaning and value of labour pain in the context of a given culture, social development and historical events. The chapter provides a description of certain, though possibly not all, specifics assigned to labour pain e.g., in France, the USA, the former Soviet Union and Great Britain. The final summary of the chapter raises the question of whether, in the 21st century, labour pain is something we should accept or avoid. The debate is perceived in the context of rapid technical developments in medicine, the explosive growth of pharmacotherapy, the widespread use of epidural anaesthesia in vaginal delivery and the desire of some women for the performance of Caesarean secttion "on demand."

Chapter Two describes the psychological and social aspects of labour pain. The introduction talks about labour pain diagnostics, emphasising the fact that the more cultural, ethnic and religious differences there are between the physician (healthcare professional) and the female patient, the less accurately the physician (or other healthcare professional) can interpret the patient's pain experience. In the light of the above, the chapter suggests that all those who facilitate a female patient's coping with labour pain should, in the first place, recognize their own feelings about pain relief and suffering. As a result, they will be better qualified to react to the patient's pain relief needs and requirements. The chapter describes in detail the psychological aspects of labour pain, such as the fear of labour pain, the woman's positive feelings about pregnancy, her previous experience with pain, her partner's participation in the birth, and the woman's confidence to cope with pain and delivery; the chapter also provides a brief summary of coping strategies.

Coping strategies are the subject of *Chapter Three.* Irrespective of the huge technical progress in medicine, a woman's right to pain relief should include the offer of non-pharmacological pain control resources and specific coping strategies. The chapter defines the concept of coping with pain and describes active cognitive and behavioural coping strategies and their effectiveness in labour pain control, emphasising the wide variety and individualized use of such strategies. The chapter further describes certain cognitive theories that affect behaviour and the selection of coping strategies. The final part of the chapter emphasises the necessity of planning labour pain coping strategies. Such a plan should include a well-designed system of prenatal preparation for the woman to learn the necessary skills.

Chapter Four offers an insight into the fear of labour pain and the treatment of such fear. The Chapter suggests that fear of labour pain is common in both women who have not yet given birth and women who have, underlining the fact that fear of labour pain is related to fear of pain in general. Due to premorbid psychological comorbidity and the growing number of everyday life stressors, women are exposed to a higher risk of fear of labour and birth, particularly if they are receiving little or no support from the close family. The chapter describes effective strategies for coping with the fear of labour pain that are based on the cooperation of a multidisciplinary midwifery team using a wide range of both pharmacological and non-pharmacological methods in supporting women with fear of pain throughout their pregnancy.

The initial part of *Chapter Five* summarises the incidence of, indications for, and certain social, cultural, economic and psychological reasons for the growing number of Caesarean sections. The chapter discusses the reasons for Caesarean delivery on maternal request, the related advantages and disadvantages and the possible assistance that should to be provided by the multidisciplinary team. The Chapter describes certain ethical dilemmas and changes in the relationship between the mother-to-be and the obstetrician where the healthcare professional needs to be skilled in, supportive psychotherapy, communication, ethics and law among other things. The chapter concludes that Caesarean delivery "on demand" requires the implementation of certain guidelines for such requests. Any solution requires the participation of the entire society as a blend of medical, social and ethical aspects are involved in a woman's request for Caesarean delivery.

Chapter number 6 focuses on the fear of childbirth. Based on a summary of results and findings of previous studies, it discusses its prevalence, aetiology, and consequences with a focus on complications that the fear of childbirth can cause during the prenatal, perinatal and postnatal period. Special attention is given to the causes of the fear of childbirth, which are divided into "hard" and psychological factors. At the end of the chapter, recommendations for practices are outlined.

The book offers an insight into labour pain in its psychological context, including the methods of coping with labour pain. The experience of labour pain is understood as an outcome of a wide spectrum of somatic and psychosocial influences. We therefore encourage multidimensional care. This book is useful for all healthcare professionals participating in the preparation of women for labour and birth, the process of labour and birth itself, and postnatal care for the mother and child. The book may benefit gynaecologists, obstetricians, anaesthesiologists, paediatricians, neonatologists and psychiatrists as well as other healthcare professionals, such as nurses, midwives, clinical psychologists, psychotherapists, social workers and physiotherapists; however, it may also be of interest to lawyers, philosophers and students of the above branches. We are aware of the fact that the various points of view taken in this book are not exhaustive; we have not covered the specifics of healthcare policy and social policy in different countries or the legal aspects of particular healthcare systems, for example. We realize that certain recommendations made in the book cannot always be implemented.

Nevertheless, we believe that the view of labour pain presented in this book might help the reader to understand the need for multidisciplinary care for women in labour, as well as multidisciplinary prenatal and postnatal care. We believe that the book may serve as a useful guide for those participating in the care and all those interested in the field.

We would like to express our thanks to the reviewers of the book, particularly to Dr. Ellena Huse, next to Ass. Prof. Dr. Thomas Meuser and Prof. Dr. Giustino Varrassi. We would like to express sincere gratitude towards Lucie Steinerová from the University of Edinburgh for helping out with the language revision. We would also like to thank all our patients, colleagues and students for their help and support in exploring the topic. Last but not least, our thanks go to both our children, Filip and Ema, who allowed us the personal experience of labour and birth and coping with labour pain and basically brought us to writing this book.

Jaroslava Raudenská and Alena Javůrková

Prague, September 2015

In: The Psychological Context of Labour Pain   ISBN: 978-1-63483-825-2
Editors: J. Raudenská and A. Javůrková © 2016 Nova Science Publishers, Inc.

Chapter 1

THE SOCIOCULTURAL CONTEXT OF THE VALUE OF LABOUR PAIN

Jaroslava Raudenská and Alena Javůrková

ABSTRACT

This chapter summarises the approach to coping with labour pain adopted in the second half of the 20th century with a particular focus on the period from the 1950s to the 1980s; in this period, the psychological understanding of labour pain among doctors and other healthcare professionals as well as among the general public was subject to major changes. At that time, two different psychological approaches to the psychology of labour pain and the general role of the woman emerged: "natural childbirth" as supported by Dick-Read, a British physician, and "psychoprophylaxis," introduced by Velvovsky, a Soviet neuropsychologist, and popularized in the West particularly by the French obstetrician Lamaze. The chapter further describes certain effects and specifics attributed to labour pain e.g., in France, the USA, the former Soviet Union and Great Britain. The chapter reflects on the dynamics of the relationship between healthcare professionals and female patients that may have influenced changes in the social meaning and value of labour pain in the context of a given culture, social development and historical events. The question is whether, at the beginning of 21st century, labour pain is something we should accept or, rather, avoid, in the context of technical developments in medicine, the explosive growth of pharmacotherapy, the widespread use of epidural anaesthesia in vaginal delivery, the desire of some women for C-section "on demand" and the changing relationship between the mother-to-be and the healthcare professional.

Keywords: coping, natural childbirth, prophylaxis, medical childbirth

INTRODUCTION

After World War II, developments in medicine allowed doctors to increasingly influence and control labour and birth; the original "expectative" approach to birth was replaced by an active medical approach. Such a major shift was facilitated by the development of pharmacology, anaesthesia, asepsis, antibiotics, sophisticated standardised procedures and advanced medical devices. In economically developed countries, childbirth was transferred to big centralized maternity hospitals that could ensure the necessary care for the mother and the child and allow for super consultation services. The aim was to secure the mother's and the child's safety and to eliminate risk. Globally, the number of maternal mortality dropped from more than 500,000 a year in 1980 to 343,000 a year in 2008. In the last 20 years, deaths have been declining at a rate of about 1.4% a year. During the late 1960s primarily postneonatal mortality declined substantially (WHO, 2014). Preventive check-ups of pregnant women were introduced together with the categories of high-risk pregnancy and pathological pregnancy. Soon, however, the above practice became the target of criticism; critical voices pointed out the excessive use of technology and pharmacotherapy at the cost of a personal, individualized and human approach to women in labour.

NATURAL CHILDBIRTH

The concept of natural childbirth was born at the end of the first half of the 20th century as a reaction to the techno-medical model and pharmacological methods of pain relief during childbirth. Natural childbirth attempts to eliminate (or minimize) pharmaceutical intervention and supports the woman's psychological needs and active participation in childbirth. The "father" of this method is Grantly Dick-Read, a British medical doctor. His books Natural Childbirth (Dick-Read, 1933) and Childbirth without Fear (Dick-Read, 1944) were published in the period of the post-war baby boom on both sides of the

Atlantic after the Second World War had slowed down population growth. His further works placed emphasis on the mother and her excellent physical condition in order to endure the stress of labour and birth. The conditions and circumstances of childbirth were therefore stipulated in the first phase, with psychological aspects added subsequently. Dick-Read stressed the patient's need to control the birth process and the pain with the help of a midwife offering empathy and acting as a coach in this stressful situation (1969). Dick-Read's version of non-medicated childbirth set an interesting trend in obstetrics at the end of the first half of 20th century (Dick-Read and Wessel, 1994). The majority of wealthy and middle-class women in Britain and the USA at that time preferred the use of pharmacology to ease labour pain. Dick-Read on the other hand believed that coping with pain by means of deep relaxation and the calm behaviour of a mother educated on the physiological aspects of pregnancy and birth was a better, safer and more satisfying way to have a child. In fact, Dick-Read believed that the pain and suffering was the product of the woman's mind rather than the body as young girls grew up believing that childbirth was a terrible experience. Education and the practice of relaxation techniques were supposed to prepare women for their fear of pain and unknown experiences. Dick-Read thought that it was fear that created muscle tension and, consequently, pain. He called this process the "fear-tension-pain cycle." Education and psychological preparation, rather than an aesthesia, were to help childbirth to once again be perceived as a normal and natural process. Until his death in 1959, Dick-Read popularized prenatal preparation courses in Great Britain and the USA. Elisabeth Bing, a physiotherapist and childbirth educator, was another natural childbirth advocate in the USA. In cooperation with Benjamin Segal she established the American Society for Psychoprophylaxis in Obstetrics (ASPO) in 1960. The organization subsequently changed its name to Lamaze International (available athttp://www.lamazeinternational.org/). The aim of ASPO was to distinguish psychoprophylaxis from Read's method of natural childbirth by emphasising the more sophisticated theoretical basis (based on Pavlov's research) and more rigorous clinical studies of psychoprophylaxis (Bing, 1994). During the Cold War, ASPO strived to disguise the Soviet origin of psychoprophylaxis. In the USA, as a result, the Russian term "psychoprophylaxis" has come to bear the name of a French obstetrician: the "Lamaze method."

PSYCHOPROPHYLAXIS

Psychoprophylaxis was developed by the Soviet psychologist I. Z. Velvovskyin 1948-1949 and was popularized by the French obstetrician Fernand Lamaze. Independently of Dick-Read's works on natural childbirth, Soviet researchers tackled similar questions on managing labour pain and came to similar conclusions. Suffering the demographic consequences of the Second World War, the Soviet Union was forced to look for ways to increase the birth rate while facing an acute lack of an aesthetics and analgesics. One of the options was the use of psychological methods to relieve pain (Michaels, 2012). After 20 years of research into the application of hypnosis during labour, Velvovsky decided to look for a more effective psychological approach to pain relief. Similarly to Dick-Read's concept of natural childbirth, educating women about the physiology of pregnancy, labour and birth helped to eliminate their fear of the unknown. The power of suggestion was used to break the negative expectation pattern; the obstetrician convinced the mothers-to-be that they should expect a painless labour and birth. Compared to Dick-Read's natural childbirth, psychoprophylaxis placed much more emphasis on the role of conscious relaxation and breathing during labour. Negative conditioning was removed by means of education and creation of new conditioned responses with the use of preparatory breathing. Psychoprophylaxis was supported by the Soviet government. In summer 1951, Fernand Lamaze visited the USSR and observed a birth using psycho-prophylaxis. Back in France, Lamaze facilitated the first French birth using psychoprophylaxis in March 1952. The hospital became a psychoprophylaxis training centre - students from all over the world learned from Lamaze (Lamaze, 1972). At the same time, the USSR promoted this method in Eastern Europe and China. In France, psychoprophylaxis was much more popular than natural childbirth. In the USA, the concept of natural childbirth was introduced first, but subsequently merged with psychoprophylaxis and the boundaries between the two methods gradually faded. Although Lamaze's followers strived to separate the two methods, the success of the Lamaze method in the USA and other English speaking countries was, to a large extent, due to Dick-Read's efforts to promote natural childbirth. In the 1950s and 1960s, a fight between the two methods broke out and some followers wanted to prove that one method was more efficient than the other. In the 1970s, the rivalry faded and the natural childbirth and Lamaze methods lowly became synonymous. While the Soviet supporters of psychoprophylaxis emphasized Pavlov's materialistic understanding of the strengths and weaknesses of a woman's nervous system as the source of labour pain, followed by left-wing French allies who, for political and ideological reasons, used the same reasoning; Dick-Read's followers in Great Britain and the USA and the more conservative

French healthcare professionals preferred a Freudian interpretation of the influence of the mind on labour pain. These obstetricians and psychologists tried to find a woman's unconscious motives and childhood experiences as the source of physical suffering during childbirth. Nevertheless, psychology rather than anaesthesiology was the key in both cases (Michaels, 2012).

Despite the gradual merger of both approaches, we would like to summarise here the basic differences between the two methods. While fear was the main disturbance factor in natural birth, psychoprophylaxis focused onnegative conditioned responses. Natural childbirth used prophylactic methods such as education, relaxation exercises, breathing and gymnastics; psychoprophylaxis used the explanation of Pavlov's responses, replacement of negative suggestions with positive ones and retraining. While natural childbirth saw the effect of preparation for labour in emotional, autonomic nerve, and muscle relaxation, psychoprophylaxis saw the effect in the replacement of negative conditioned responses with positive ones. In preparation for labour under natural childbirth the pregnant woman's focus was on active relaxation and psychological preparation with slow relaxing breathing; psychoprophylaxis prepared the woman for active cooperation using fast activating breathing to divert attention with the aim of reaching a painless labour.

FURTHER DEVELOPMENT OF NATURAL CHILDBIRTH AND PSYCHOPROFYLAXIS

Even though they underwent prenatal preparation, women in France, the USA and other countries experienced labour pain. They often felt like failures and were assigned some sort of emotional disturbance to account for the labour pain. For psychoprophylaxis supporters, a woman in labour who experienced pain and expressed it with pain behaviour (screaming, crying, grimaces, etc.), or requested anaesthesiology was a failure. The woman was the only one to blame while the limited effects of the method were not an option. Psychoprophylaxis supporters assigned the woman's partial or complete failure to two potential reasons: external causes connected with the application of the method (noise in the delivery room, hostile staff, insufficient instructions and education) or the woman's internal causes (Karmel, 1959). The obstetrician, psychologist or birth educator responsible for evaluating the female patient's birth behaviour often explained the woman's failure by the "sensitivity" of her cortical balance. French mothers in the 1950s were often sad about disappointing their obstetricians as well as themselves. They felt responsible for the failure (i.e., experiencing pain during labour) and hoped to do better next time. In the 1960s, the representatives of ASPO agreed with the French that labour pain was primarily psychogenic. At the same time, American women accepted pain as normal part of natural childbirth. Although obstetricians did not consider childbirth successful if the woman experienced pain, American women evaluated their psychoprophylactic childbirth as successful, even if they felt strong pain. In France, where psychoprophylaxis gained much more popularity, there were very high expectations for the absence of pain. In the USA however, where prophylaxis was preceded by the influence of Dick-Read's theory of "childbirth without fear" for nearly two decades, women did not try to eliminate pain but rather looked for tools to manage it. What is interesting is that the thinking of American women in this period was very close to the understanding of Soviet healthcare professionals after 1956, when de-Stalinization led to a more open discussion about medical research and clinical practice methods (Michaels, 2012). Eventually, voices were raised by Soviet obstetricians claiming the limits of psychoprophylaxis. They calmed down the excitement about the anaesthetic effect of psychoprophylaxis as a virtual remedy for labour pain and, instead, stressed the method's value as a means of support. Later, the training practically disappeared from Soviet midwifery and was replaced by an ignorant and arrogant approach to labour pain and suffering (Michaels, 2012). Unlike Soviet women, French women in the 1970s got the opportunity to protest again the idealization of psychoprophylaxis in childbirth in the new atmosphere characterized by feminism, Planned Parenthood and the legalization of abortion. Unlike the previous generation blaming themselves for pain (i.e., failure during childbirth), the new generation of women directed their anger towards the obstetricians, midwives, hospital staff in general, the maternity hospitals' set up, organization and regulations, and the limited effects of the method. Women's disappointment was most often connected with the lack of relief from pain promised by psychoprophylaxis. In addition, women were displeased when, regardless of their requests, hospital staff refused to give them medication to relieve pain. Thus, the 1970s can be seen as a period in which French women fought against the narrow definition of an "ideal female patient" and requested pharmacological pain relief while refusing personal guilt for their inability to use psychoprophylaxis as their only tool for coping with pain. While the entitlement to drugs was part of the fight for rights and freedoms in France; in the USA, which was inclined to strongly medicated childbirth, feminism and feminine authority were confirmed by the refusal of drugs. In the atmosphere of rising feminist consciousness of the 1970s labour without anaesthesia meant resistance to the power of obstetricians for American women. They called labour and birth "hard work" and refused to suppress or avoid pain; rather, they accepted labour as a challenge. Pain was accepted as a normal part of the process of childbirth and success was seen as coping with pain as opposed to not feeling pain. A number of educated middle-class American women and their partners perceived significance assigned to pain and elevated natural childbirth to a kind of ritual. By the 1980s, the idea that psychoprophylaxis would guarantee the elimination of pain was finally abandoned even by those American healthcare professionals who had previously protected the Lamaze method. Unlike the early Lamaze activists, the new generation of healthcare professionals confirmed the belief of many American mothers: psychoprophylaxis can help a patient cope with pain rather than removing pain.

OTHER FOLLOWERS OF NATURAL CHILDBIRTH

Rather than directly eliminating fear or pain, other natural childbirth followers focused on the mother's maturity, improvement of delivery room conditions, creating an environment of empathy, and respect for the mother's needs and wishes. Since the 1960s, Sheila Kitzinger, a British social anthropologist, has encouraged in her lectures and multiple publications the pregnant woman's responsibility and strength to give birth naturally. She also believes that women who do not have a high-risk pregnancy should have a chance to have their baby at home to their own benefit. Her work focused on the "elimination of fear of the baby's passing through and leaving the mother's body" by means of practicing relaxation and special positions during childbirth. She did not stress coping with pain, but childbirth as a form of a woman's growth and maturation (Kitzinger, 1996). In the 1960s, Frederick Leboyer, a French obstetrician, popularized, in his publication Birth Without Violence (Leboyer, 1975), gentle and natural childbirth, particularly the practice of immersing newborn infants in a small tub of warm water - known as the "Leboyer bath" - to help ease the baby's transition from the womb to the outside world. He also advocated that the newborn be laid on its mother's stomach and allowed to bond, instead of being taken away for tests. He criticised maternity wards that were full of stressors for both the woman and the child. In his opinion, the strange hospital environment, impersonal approach of the hospital staff, noise and lighting all contributed to the woman's anxiety during childbirth. Newborn babies scream because they are held upside down by the lower extremities, exposed to light and cold, and the umbilical cord is cut. Leboyer also focused on the psychological preparation of the mother for bonding with her child, on educating the mother on how to approach her child and on educating obstetricians on their approach to labour and birth (quietness, gentleness, calmness, patience, focus on the mother, placing the child on its mother's belly with fingers toward the axilla, cutting the umbilical cord only after it stopped pulsating, etc.). The idea of "gentle childbirth" was further developed by Michel Odent, a French obstetrician, in his book "Natural Childbirth" (Odent, 2007) at the end of the 1970s and the beginning of the 1980s. He understands childbirth as a natural expression of a woman's body needing no external intervention. He believes that respecting the pregnant woman's basic needs is the first and utmost prerequisite for successful childbirth; these may include undisturbed peace, warmth, intimacy and safety. Odent creates an environment in which a woman can lead the labour and birth process freely in her own way and pace and in which anything is possible. If she wants to scream, she screams; if she wants to have the baby in darkness or wants to have her other children around, she may have that; if, just before partum, she wants to walk around the room or be carried to water in a pool and give birth in the water, she is encouraged to use her own way.

MODERN REFLECTIONS ON NATURAL CHILDBIRTH

In the middle of the 20th century, supporters of Read's method and psychoprophylaxis claimed that women did not need to suffer pain during childbirth. Refuting the idea of pain as a normal and natural part of the childbirth process, they saw the key to pain in the woman's brain. Labour pain was stripped of its social value or biological function and was perceived as a test of the woman's mental health. Gradually, however, a new opinion prevailed: labour pain is a natural feature of childbirth; in the USA, the presence of labour pain became a test of the woman's strength or spiritual depth rather than mental weakness. This "idealized picture" of childbirth was not as popular in France as many French women were deeply disappointed after being promised "pain free childbirth" by the promoters of psychoprophylaxis. The French obstetricians' reluctance to ease labour pain using pharmacological methods was in contradiction to the motive of American women: they refused pain relief drugs as a gesture of rebellion against the American obstetricians' authority (Michaels, 2012). At the end of the 1980s, the benefits of natural childbirth and prophylaxis were revaluated, but almost no studies were available to prove the effectiveness of both basic methods of coping with fear and pain, while the existing studies contained methodological errors (Beck and Hall, 1978).

In the 1980s and in subsequent years, an individualized approach to the mother-to-be and demedicalization of childbirth were the main trends of natural childbirth; medication was only called for after all natural non-pharmacological methods were exhausted. The detechnization of childbirth was also highlighted; technology was only to be used in a non-invasive way. Continuity of care is another important factor; ideally, a single midwife and a single medical doctor should take care of the mother-to-be throughout the preconception period, pregnancy, and childbirth and post-natal period. The importance of education has kept its validity; only a well-informed mother-to-be, knowledgeable of all available options, advantages, disadvantages and risks, can take a pro-active part in the decision making (selection of the maternity hospital, childbirth method, childbirth plan, etc.). Humanisation of the environment, intimacy, privacy during labour and the presence of partner and family also fall among the most important requirements. In a safe environment, qualified medical and nursing care is available at any time, if needed. Healthcare professionals are expected to take an open, accepting, accommodating and supportive approach to the woman. Natural childbirth should take place in a quiet, calm, semi-dark environment and the woman should feel free and should be able to move freely and change position. Communication between the woman, her partner and the healthcare professionals should take place on an equal level, in partnership.

MEDICAL OR NATURAL CHILDBIRTH?

In view of recent technical developments in modern medicine, the question of coping with labour pain has triggered a lively public discussion. The medical approach to childbirth and pain management referred to in the introduction to this chapter recognises a number of risks involved in pregnancy and childbirth and promotes childbirth led by a healthcare professional and pain management using pharmacology. Proven medical interventions and nursing care are used to prevent any problems from arising. Such childbirth may suit women who rely on the achievements of modern medicine and the powerful authority of doctors and other hospital staff rather than their natural power. Such women believe that experienced medical doctors and other healthcare professionals in a technically well-equipped delivery room guarantee safe childbirth and allow the women to waive their own responsibility for the birth. The current generation of mothers in economically developed countries appreciate, also thanks to their doctors' recommendations, effective pharmacological pain relief methods even during spontaneous vaginal childbirth. Many women in developed countries expect that modern medicine should free them from all sorts of risks, suffering and pain (Howard, 2003). However, such expectations are unrealistic.

On the other hand, childbirth is connected with dehumanisation and a loss of meaning of pain during labour and the woman's right to choose natural childbirth without medical interventions and pharmacotherapy. Childbirth and its accompanying pain are perceived as a natural physiological process that most women can naturally handle and medical and nursing care should only create optimal conditions for a smooth natural process. Medicine should not try to control or accelerate the process of childbirth or to intervene, but rather supervise its safety. Natural childbirth may be the choice of women who are used to taking an active approach to their own health and refusing the role of passive patients. Such women may believe that natural labour mechanisms, including pain, have a deeper meaning, feel their own responsibility for the childbirth, and trust they can cope with labour pain.

CONCLUSION

The right balance between pharmacotherapeutic, non-pharmacotherapeutic and psychological approaches to coping with pain should be found while respecting the woman's needs and wishes. A heated discussion among experts and the public about the reasonability of natural childbirth celebrating the maturity of the woman and mother versus a "safe" medicated childbirth using pharmacology for pain relief demonstrates that the meaning and value of labour pain in its cultural and historical context is a highly sensitive topic.

In: The Psychological Context of Labour Pain   ISBN: 978-1-63483-825-2
Editors: J. Raudenská and A. Javůrková © 2016 Nova Science Publishers, Inc.

Chapter 2

PSYCHOLOGICAL ASPECTS OF LABOUR PAIN

Jaroslava Raudenská, Jana Amlerová and Alena Javůrková

ABSTRACT

This chapter focuses on the psychological and social aspects of labour pain. The introduction describes methods of labour pain diagnostics and the evaluation of the woman's pain experience by healthcare professionals. As nociceptive stimuli in labour pain are interpreted centrally using the interaction of a wide spectrum of emotional, motivational, social, cultural and cognitive factors specific to the woman in labour, this is reflected in the general diagnostics and in the concept of unique individual experiences of labour pain. The chapter describes in detail certain psychological aspects of labour pain such as fear of labour pain, the woman's positive feelings about pregnancy, previous experience with pain, the partner's participation in childbirth, and the woman's confidence to cope with pain and labour; the chapter also provides a brief summary of coping strategies.

Keywords: pain diagnostics, psychological and social aspects

INTRODUCTION

Pain during labour is a subjective response that is not related to any pathology. From the timeframe perspective, labour pain is considered acute pain. Pain during labour is a practically universal experience and women expect childbirth to be a painful experience (Fillingim, 2005). The pain is caused by strong uterine contractions in forcing out the foetus and the pressure of the baby on the soft and hard tissues of the birth canal; in addition, various micro traumas occur in the birth canal. The first stage of labour starts with regular uterine contractions causing dilation of the cervix and ends with full dilation of the cervix. According to modern textbooks, the first stage takes about 6-7 hours, which is less than previously, particularly due to medical childbirth. The pain is visceral, dull. In the latent phase, the pain radiates to T 11-12; during the active phase with further progress, the pain affects an area from T 10 up to L 1 (McDonald and Noback, 2003). The intensity of pain gradually increases with the dilation of the cervix. At the end of stage one, the baby's head is descending to the pelvis, causing pressure on the lumbosacral plexus and consequent pain in segments L 2 - S 1. In the final phase, pain is more frequently connected with contractions. The second stage of labour starts with the full dilation and disappearance of the cervix and ends with the expulsion of the baby. This stage takes about 5-20 minutes. During the progression, the baby's head must rotate. Pain during the second stage of labour is somatic and sharp, caused by pressure on the pelvic diaphragm, vagina and perineum. The baby continues descending towards the vaginal opening and the entire vaginal canal continues to stretch. Final passage of the head through the middle pelvis causes stretching of the tissues of the middle and lower vagina and extension of the vaginal opening. Painful stimuli from these areas are carried by the pudendal nerve to segments S 2 – S 4. The third stage of labour starts when the baby is born and ends with the delivery of the placenta and amniotic sac; this stage takes 5-30 minutes. The third stage is accompanied by pain relief. After the placenta is expelled, uterine receptors receive stimulation and the uterine involution starts. Treatment of injuries suffered during labour may cause certain additional pain. The post-partum period, sometimes called the fourth stage of labour, is the period of the first two hours after birth. Spontaneous pain is no longer perceived at this stage. This period is important for the feeling of satisfaction with labour and the pain experienced, and the bonding and early connection between the mother and the baby.

ACQUIRING INFORMATION ABOUT PAIN DURING LABOUR

Apart from the senses, other aspects of labour pain include emotions, evaluation, behaviour and social processes. A two-directional causality is at work here. If a female patient experiences labour pain, she will always have an emotional reaction to the pain; she will have certain ideas about pain, herself, the world and her future, she will evaluate, and she will behave in a specific way. The diagnostics of labour pain focuses on retrospective observation of pain behaviour (Bonica, 1990). The validity of data acquired during labour may be limited (Baker, Ferguson, Roach and Dawson, 2001). Recollection of pain may be vivid, but not always accurate (Niven and Murphy-Black, 2000). In some women, the memory of labour and labour pain may provoke an intensive negative response which may relate to memories of the healthcare professionals' care, feeling of safety and self-confidence to cope with the pain and labour (Waldenström, 2004).

The Sensory Component of Pain

Concerning the sensory component of pain, diagnostics focuses on the *intensity, quality and location* of pain. The most frequent way of measuring labour pain is by means of verbal statements. If a woman in labour claims that she is experiencing pain, such pain is always considered real (McCaffery and Pasero, 1999). If the intensity of pain is the subject of evaluation, a statement may not always fully represent the emotional, motivational and socio-cultural aspects. A Visual Analogue Scale, VAS (100 mm horizontal line) is used to establish the intensity of pain. The outermost left-hand point of the continuum says "no pain," the right-hand point says "worst pain I can imagine." Labour pain is usually between 64 and 86 mm on VAS (Sheiner, K., Sheiner, E., Shoham-Vardi, Mazor and Katz, 1999), i.e., high or very high intensity pain. Limits to VAS are caused by the woman's position during labour; she cannot record the intensity of pain. Some women cannot perceive absolute or normative values of both ends of the scale in repeated measurements of pain intensity − it is necessary to consider possible intrasubjective changes in maximum values and the effects of medication (Wewers and Lowe, 1990). The interpretation of the right-hand side of the continuum of the scale depends on the woman's previous experience with pain. Healthy, young primiparas may evaluate the same pain as more intense than secundiparas or a woman who has previously experienced pain (Lowe, 1996). Other options for measuring the intensity of labour pain are numerical scales, iconic scales and verbal scales. An example of a verbal scale is the Index Present Pain (IPP) attached to the short form of the McGill Pain Questionnaire (SF-MPQ, Melzack 1987). The intensity of labour pain in primiparae and multiparae using IPP was higher than in patients with chronic backache, oncological pain in non-terminal stages, postherpetic neuralgia, phantom pains, toothache or arthritic pain (Melzack, Taenzer, Feldman and Kinch, 1981). On the IPP scale, level 5 pain (unbearable) was reported by 25% of all primipara and 9% of all multipara mothers. Certain women who marked labour pain with level 4 and 5 intensity avoided verbal expression of the numerical value (4 – severe pain, 5 – unbearable pain), as the positive experience of having a baby prevented them from using negative words. Higher intensities of pain than during labour were only reported by patients with acute pain after finger amputation or patients with causalgia (Melzack and Katz, 1999).

Measuring the intensity of pain by means of a medical doctor's estimate is useful if the woman in labour cannot provide her own evaluation due to time or procedural restraints or if she lacks the necessary cognitive or language skills. There is a difference between the evaluation of labour pain intensity by a doctor and that by the mother (Brown, Campbell and Kurtz, 1989). The bigger the cultural, ethnic or religious difference between the doctor and the patient, the less precisely the doctor can interpret the pain experience of the mother (Sheiner, E., Sheiner, E. K., Hershkovitz, Mazor, Katz and Shoham-Vardi, 2000). For these reasons, all those helping the patient cope with labour pain should be aware of their own feelings about pain and suffering in order to be able to perceive a patient's requirements for pain relief (Raudenska, Amlerova and Javurkova, 2014).

The *location* of pain may be acquired by drawing the painful points (Pasero and McCaffery, 2011). The *quality* of pain may be measured using SF-MPQ. Women often describe labour pain as oppressive, burning, stabbing, acute, cramping, pulsating, sharp or shooting. On the emotional scale, pain is often described as exhausting, intense and bothering (Brown, Campbell and Kurtz, 1989). Women who reported lower back pain during labour described the pain as pressure, oppressive, stabbing, sharp, burning, and, from the emotional point of view as tiring and bothering (Melzack and Schaffelberg, 1987).

The Emotional Component of Pain

It is often difficult for the patient to differentiate emotions from the sensory component of pain. Evaluation of the emotional component of pain is closely related to the cultural origin of the obstetrician and the midwifery team and their attitude to and beliefs about means of easing the woman's pain, anxiety, fear and suffering and supporting her. Questionnaires and inventories are used retrospectively to measure anxiety, fear and depression in labour pain. For example the Spielberger's state-trait anxiety inventory (STAI), the Beck Depression Inventory (BDI), the Beck Anxiety Inventory (BAI), the Edinburgh Postnatal Depression Scale (EPDS) or the Delivery Fear Scale.

The Behavioural Component of Pain

Rating scales or video records are used to observe behaviour. The aim is to determine what the patient does and how she behaves when in pain. Most women in labour, when experiencing intensive pain, look for help and display strong pain behaviour (wrinkling, facial expressions, grimaces, vocal expression, etc.). The healthcare professional or partner labour may support or reduce such behaviour. The Present Behavioral Intensity Scale (PBIS) (Bonnel and Boureau, 1985) allows for observation of pain behaviour during labour (breathing patterns, movement reactions, agitation). However, the average values of pain behaviour observed by the doctor were 1.2 points lower than the verbal evaluation of pain intensity given by the woman in labour (Melzack and Katz, 1999). Pain is a complex and subjective experience; thus, little concordance can be expected between various methods of pain measurement, pain behaviour or various observers.

The Cognitive Component of Pain

Methods of cognitive processing of pain should test the patient's opinion of pain, schema of pain explanation, coping with pain, self-awareness and self-evaluation. It is possible to use questionnaires to evaluate the cognitive area of chronic pain. The questionnaires focus on negative, unrealistic or catastrophic opinions, beliefs, thoughts and schemas activated by the experience of pain. For example the Wijma Delivery Expectancy Questionnaire (W-DEQ) and Childbirth Self-Efficacy Inventory (CBSEI), the Women's Views of Birth

Labour Satisfaction Questionnaire (WOMBLSQ) or Sullivan´s the Pain Catastrophizing Scale.

SOCIAL FACTORS

The experience of pain during labour is highly individual and depends on the relationships between biopsychosocial factors. *Increased intensity of pain* is generally associated with first time labour and birth in the woman's life, lower age, lower level of education, general fear of pain, insensitive approach of the hospital staff, ignorance of the woman's needs during labour and unresolved psychological disturbance. *Lower pain intensity* is generally connected with attending prenatal classes, a higher socio-economic status, the woman's higher level of education and age, her willingness to breastfeed, the support and sensitive approach of the staff and a safe environment (Melzack, 1984; Tournaire and Theau-Yonneau, 2007; Waldenström, Hildingsson, Rubertsson and Rådestad, 2004) (Read in detail in chapter 5).

The extent to which a woman in labour considers her environment safe is closely related to her personality and personal experience of social relationships, her communication style, the method of childbirth in the given country, the quality of support provided by the healthcare staff and their beliefs about whether, and how to ease pain. No differences in the subjective intensity of pain during labour were observed between e.g., Afro-American and White American women (Winsberg and Greenlick, 1967), Australian women and women born in Italy (Pesce, 1987), Dutch women and American women (Senden, Wetering, Eskes, Biewrkens, Laube and Pitkin, 1988), women from Kuwait, Palestine and Bedouin women (Harrison, 1991), Jewish and Bedouin women (Sheiner K., Sheiner, E., Shoham-Vardi, Mazor and Katz, 1999) or between American women and Korean women living in the US. There are no studies comparing the *emotional dimension of pain* of various cultures and ethnic groups. *Pain behaviour* in various cultural and subcultural groups may differ as it results from the acquired pattern of a woman's expected behaviour in labour. As a girl grows to become a woman, women's stories give her an understanding of what happens with a woman's body and with pain during labour and birth and how women usually behave. A higher intensity of pain may relate to the pregnant woman's *lower level of education* (Weisenberg and Caspi, 1989). Mechanisms that could explain these associations include variations in behavioural and environmental risk factors by educational status, differences in occupational factors, differences in access to and utilisation of health services, and adaptation to stress. Consequently, education may change the influence of the environment, culture and reaction to pain. However, even a woman that has undergone preparation for labour and pain may be caught off guard. The important thing is the general *approach to labour pain relief* in the patient's environment/country of residence. For example, the following two beliefs are quite common in the US: labour pain should be eased as soon as possible and labour pain and stress related to labour and birth is best avoided by planning a CS (Waters, 1998). Compared to Dutch women for instance, American women expect labour to be much more painful and request more medication and invasive methods to cope with labour pain. Dutch women, on the other hand, understand labour as a natural process and most of them do not require any special interventions (Christiaens, Verhaeghe and Bracke, 2010). Nevertheless, the intensity of labour pain is not the primary factor determining *satisfaction with labour and birth* across cultures (Hodnett, 2002). Satisfaction means coping with pain rather than eliminating it, being able to influence, to a certain extent, the labour process and result, feeling safe and experiencing verbal support provided by the medical staff.

PSYCHOLOGICAL FACTORS

Fear of Labour Pain

Women with irrational fear of pain generally show a lower tolerance to pain. Behaviour aimed towards avoiding pain is connected with anxiety (Lowe, 2002; Saisto and Halmesmäki, 2003; Saisto, Kaaja, Ylikorkala and Halmesmäki, 2001). Anxiety in pregnancy and labour may result from conflicts during pregnancy, social and financial insecurity or lack of information (Saisto, Salmela-Aro, Nurmi and Halmesmäki, 2001b). Anxious women more frequently require epidural analgesia and Caesarean section and report higher intensity of pain and fear of pain and worse cooperation of healthcare personnel during labour (Bussche, Crombez, Eccleston and Sullivan, 2007; Rouhe, Salmela-Aro, Halmesmäki and Saisto, 2009; Tsui, Pang, Melender, Xu, Lau and Lejny, 2006; Waldenström, Hildingsson and Ryding, 2006). Anxiety in general applies to pregnancy, labour and birth, the result of the birth process, consequences for the woman and other issues. Thanks to the release of endogenous opioids initiated by anxiety during pregnancy and labour, pain is better tolerated. Increased anxiety during labour, however, is related to increased pain intensity. The increased secretion of catecholamine may increase nociception from the pelvis and strengthen the perception of nociceptive stimuli on the cortical level (Lowe, 1996), thus extending the first stage of labour (Alehagen, Wijma, K. and Wijma, B., 2006). Both fear and anxiety also lead to muscle tension and thus increase pain (Chapter 4 provides further information on the fear of labour pain).

A Positive Approach

A woman's positive approach to pregnancy may increase her tolerance of pain during labour as pain is perceived as a positive rather than a destructive force. There is a correlation between a woman's longing for pregnancy and children and a lower intensity of pain during labour and the effective use of coping strategies (Niven and Gijsbers, 1996). Patients whose pregnancy was unplanned or illegal or those whose reaction to conception was ambivalent or negative can report a higher intensity of labour pain. Furthermore, women with premature or induced labour may report a higher intensity of labour pain, which may be related to the emotional or endocrine preparedness of the woman.

Previous Experience

Previous experience with pain gives the mother-to-be an opportunity to create experience-based coping skills and attitudes to pain and have a positive impact on the unique interpretation of nociception during labour. For most healthy primiparas, labour is their first experience of acute pain (Niven and Gijsbers, 1984). Higher tolerance and lower intensity of pain is therefore expected in multiparas, women with previous experience of pain in general, older women and women with higher levels of education. Women who suffered intense lower back pain during pregnancy, overweight women or those with a large foetus may report a higher intensity of pain during labour. The experience of subjectively unbearable pain together with loss of control and dissatisfaction with ways of coping with labour may result in postnatal emotional disorders, particularly postnatal depression or posttraumatic stress disorder (PTSD) (Edworthy, Chasey and Williams, 2008; Sawyer and Ayers, 2009). These may weaken the woman's mental health and negatively affect her early relationship with the child, causing fear of future pregnancy and negatively affecting her sexual life with her partner. Women who expected a painless labour or manageable pain, but, once confronted with pain, requested epidural analgesia, may feel personal failure.

Birth Partner

The relationship between the mother and the child's father and his presence during birth plays an important role in the intensity of pain experienced in labour. With men entering the delivery room, another step was taken towards the humanisation of labour and birth process. The father's presence during birth may have both positive and negative effects. With some women, the intensity of pain increased with the presence of their husband. Other women, who had been supported by their partners throughout the whole pregnancy and childbirth, experienced lower intensity of pain in labour, required less pain relief and the labour was shorter with fewer complications. Modern society expects fathers to be present at birth and this presence is seen as a benchmark for the measurement of fulfilment of their male and fatherhood roles.

The Woman's Self-Efficacy and Coping Strategies

Healthy women delivering their baby at term and who are confident that they can cope with both the labour and the pain (the "self-efficacy" concept) (Bandura, 1997; Lowe, 2002), and women who have been educated about coping strategies in prenatal preparation courses have a good chance of experiencing lower intensity of pain during labour (Christiaens and Bracke, 2007). A woman's low confidence in her coping with pain relates to her irrational fear of labour and pain, higher levels of adopted powerlessness, an external locus of control and a generally lower self-esteem and self-confidence. A woman's trust in her ability to succeed and cope with labour and pain increases with experience, e.g., in multiparas.

Women reported relaxation, attention distraction and focusing, imagination and deep breathing techniques as effective coping strategies in dealing with labour pain. Low self-confidence in dealing with stressful situations in general (low self-efficacy) was a significant predictor of pain intensity in the first stage of labour and birth, followed by fear of pain, anxiety about the labour process and result, previous experience with non-gynaecological pain, cervical dilation, contraction frequency, menstrual pain, the woman's prenatal weight and the newborn baby's height and weight. The number of coping strategies used correlates with the intensity of pain (Niven and Gijsbers, 1996). Women in labour use coping strategies that they are familiar with and which they are used to applying in other stressful situations (see more about coping strategies in Chapter 3).

CONCLUSION

The level of pain experienced in labour is unique for each woman and may be affected by somatic factors, the psychosocial specifics of the woman, cultural beliefs, birthing environment and the healthcare provided. It is therefore advisable to work with women suffering from unreasonable anxiety, depression or significant psychological and social problems as early as the prenatal period.

In: The Psychological Context of Labour Pain   ISBN: 978-1-63483-825-2
Editors: J. Raudenská and A. Javůrková © 2016 Nova Science Publishers, Inc.

Chapter 3

COPING WITH LABOUR PAIN

Jaroslava Raudenská and Alena Javůrková

ABSTRACT

While some people adapt well to pain, others do not. The same applies to coping with labour pain. This chapter draws on the literature on coping with both acute pain and labour pain. The chapter starts with a definition of coping and focuses primarily on active coping strategies (both cognitive and behavioural) and their effectiveness in coping with labour pain. The chapter emphasises the strengthening of strategies that are more adaptive in coping with labour pain. The number and types of strategies used in coping with labour pain are individual and varied. The chapter further describes certain cognitive theories that understand the purpose of our behaviour as a key predictor in selecting coping strategies. Finally, the chapter reconfirms the necessity of planning coping strategies in order to cope with labour pain and provides a summary of the influence of psychological knowledge on the improvement of women's prenatal education.

Keywords: coping strategy, cognition, cognitive theory

INTRODUCTION

Labour pain is generally described as very strong acute pain, the intensity of which increases throughout the labour and birth process. Although women may find the meaning and depth of their own femininity and transition to motherhood and parenthood in labour pain, suitable coping strategies should be searched for. In general, one can distinguish between pharmacological and non-pharmacological coping strategies (Henry and Nand, 2004). The pharmacological approach includes systemic analgesia (oral, intramuscular, intravenous, inhalation) and regional analgesia methods. These are components of medical childbirth. Pharmacological methods of labour pain relief in spontaneous vaginal childbirth raise questions about the meaning and value of labour pain. While one part of the population requests intensive pharmacological pain relief, another part of the population insists on a return to natural childbirth (closely described in Chapter 1). For example, the use of epidural analgesia in spontaneous vaginal birth prevails in economically developed countries. If, however, such procedures were offered to women e.g., in poor regions of Africa, they would definitely choose it (Lewis and Harris, 2010). The use of epidural analgesia as one of the pharmacological methods of coping with labour pain in spontaneous vaginal childbirth has grown significantly. It was used by 22% of American women in 1981, 65% in 1997 and around 75% in 2009 (Michaels, 2012). Around the year 2000, the method was used by 50% of women in France, 23% in Great Britain and 45% in Canada (Fanning, Campion, Collins et al., 2008; Ruppen, Derry, McQuay and Moore, 2006). The situation in different maternity wards may, however, vary. Non-pharmacological methods include psychological, alternative medicine (acupuncture, acupressure, homeopathy), manual, bioelectromagnetic (e.g., Transcutaneous Electrical Nerve Stimulation, TENS), and physical and alternative medication (e.g., aromatherapy) methods (Chez and Jonas, 1997). The psychological approach uses prenatal preparation, partner and family support, the empathy and support of healthcare professionals including placebos, a safe environment (Simkim and O'Hara, 2002), and specific psychological methods.

A recent major examination of reviews on the efficacy and safety of labour pain interventions found strong evidence that epidural injections; combined spinal epidurals and an inhaled analgesic are effective in managing of labour pain, but all are associated with adverse effects. Methods that may work are immersion in water, relaxation, acupuncture, massage, local anesthetic nerve block and nonopioid drugs. These methods can assist in managing labour pain with relatively few adverse effects. In most cases, women did report satisfaction with pain relief, but evidence was mainly limited to individual trials. Little evidence that nonpharmacologic approaches are effective was found. Effectiveness of hypnosis, biofeedback, sterile water injection, aromatherapy, (TENS), and the use of parenteral opioids is unclear because there is too little high-quality evidence. That is why we need further trials of nonpharmacologic pain management methods and to tailor labour pain relief methods used to an individual woman's wishes, needs and individual circumstances (Jones, Othman and Dowswell, et al., 2012).

COPING

The term "coping" has two meanings: a reaction to a stressful event irrespective of its efficiency in relieving or eliminating the stressor, and an elimination of a stressor or a relief in reaction to stress. Whenever an individual is exposed to a stressful event (pain, fear of pain), he/she will react in a certain way. This reaction may have a positive or negative effect. When researching the patterns and types of reactions, individual cognitive evaluation of the meaning of each reaction has to be taken into consideration. In order to effectively cope with pain, we need to know the cause of the pain and the meaning of pain for the given individual. The understanding of and coping with pain depends on a personal understanding of the meaning of pain in an individual's story and on the sociocultural and economic context of the individual (Winterowd, Beck and Gruener, 2003). Coping with, predictability of, and meaning of pain are demonstrated in the following two short case reports: "Anna, a primipara, started feeling pain in her lower abdomen when she was at home. She had the following thoughts: "Is it a sign of labour? Am I giving birth? The pain is terrible, overwhelming. I cannot bear it any longer." She imagined the pain gradually taking hold of her entire body and with this picture in mind she felt the pain with increased intensity. She fell into despair, lay down and started crying." Why did she feel so miserable? It was not just the intensity of the pain; it was what she thought of the pain and how she behaved, i.e., the meaning she ascribed to the pain. She interpreted her pain as unbearable: she considered herself helpless. Her negative thinking had a significant impact on her general attitude to pain. "Alice, a multipara, felt a dulling and burning pain in her lower back with approaching labour. She thought: 'I feel pain, yet I know the pain is going to be even bigger. What can I do? I will try to hold my breath for a while and think about something else. It really is painful. But the pain may subside if I try to cope with it. I must focus on relaxing my body; I'll try a massage and I'll think about something nice to endure the pain. The pain is certainly not so bad that I need to ask for an epidural. I need to wait and calm down; my husband supports me.' " Compared to Anna, Alice was much more realistic about the pain. Similarly to Anna, the subjective intensity of her pain was high, but her line of thinking was different. She focused on coping with the pain; she realized what she could do, e.g., relax and distract her attention from the pain. The way she thought about the pain helped her cope with the pain in a much better way.

One concept of adaptation strategies in acute pain makes a distinction between active and passive coping (Ramirez-Maestre, Esteve and Lopez, 2008), i.e., active or passive reaction. Coping is positively influenced if an individual is able to remove the cause of pain or participate in soothing the pain. Active coping using cognitive and behavioural techniques is connected with a lower intensity of pain and depression and better self-efficacy (Stevens, Watt-Watson and Gibbins, 2003). It requires responsibility and a pro-active approach to coping with pain. Passive coping (avoiding pain and escaping using e.g., a demand for Caesarean section) is connected with a higher level of stress and emotional distress, higher intensity of pain and lower self-efficacy in both a short-term and long-term perspective (Büssing, Ostermann, Neugebauer and Heusser, 2010). The patient does not take responsibility and requests responsibility from the outside – from the "almighty" doctor, technology or drugs. Certain strategies are hard to be categorized as passive strategies as active compliance is always required for e.g., the use of drugs or an intervention. A completely passive coping strategy where no effort or decision is needed on the patient's part is difficult to imagine. Coping strategies may be measured by means of self-perception tools (questionnaires, inventories).

ACTIVE COPING STRATEGIES AND THEIR EFFECTIVENESS

A wide variety of cognitive and behavioural techniques are available to use. Cognitive techniques include changes of cognition using one's imagination, cognitive reframing, cognitive restructuring, self-instruction and distraction mechanisms (distracting attention). Behavioural strategies influence coping with pain by means of activities, e.g., relaxation techniques, breathing exercises, biofeedback or hypnosis. The self-instruction technique includes either coping with pain (emphasis on enduring pain) or reinterpretation of pain (denying negative aspects of pain and focusing on positive aspects). Effective coping with acute pain involves focusing on pain and diverting attention from pain. *Attention distraction* is based on attention processing. The more an individual needs to concentrate on a task designed to distract attention, the more pain relief is achieved. The more the mother-to-be is able to distract her attention from the pain, the more effective the technique. Attention distraction strategies may be passive (attention is redirected elsewhere, e.g., pictures from holidays) or active (i.e., tasks that compete with pain, e.g., countdown). Subjective reduction of pain perception by distracting attention from pain is an example of how cognitive processes may influence the modulation of pain, under the condition that the intensity of the pain is not too high (Raudenska, Amlerova and Javurkova, 2014). *Acceptance* is a strategy, which is expected to increase pain tolerance more than the attention distraction technique. In a study by Kohl, Rief and Glombiewski (2013), the acceptance of pain resulted in the tolerance of experimental pain increasing more than through cognitive restructuring. Unlike attention distraction, however, acceptance could not reduce the intensity of experimental pain as much. Searching for information, education, solutions and problem reframing techniques used in preparation for labour work particularly mitigate uneasiness and anxiety. Positive interpretation of labour pain allows for the perception of the experience of labour pain as a positive reinforcement of the meaning of life (and, consequently, congruence with the labour situation), and for the belief that labour pain is manageable. Imagination means creating mental pictures that are incompatible with the pain or alter the experience of pain. Imagination reduced the intensity of acute pain in comparison with a control group that did not work with imagination (Fernandez and Turk, 1989). Hypnosis in women reduced fear, tension and pain during labour and the need for pharmacological analgesia (Gentz, 2001; Mairs, 1995). The effect increased with the simultaneous practice of auto relaxation. Biofeedback allows the patient to receive feedback on physiological information that she is not usually aware of. Combined with relaxation techniques for coping with pain, biofeedback reduces the intensity of pain and use of pharmacotherapy (Bernat, Wooldridge, Marecki and Snell, 1992), provided the delivery room staff is willing to use the technique.

COGNITION, BEHAVIOUR AND COPING

People behave differently in various situations based on their cognitive processes, particularly evaluation, expectation and motivation. The selection of coping strategies is related to the expected (i.e., successful) result, achieving the goal and the value of the goal. The cognitive theories described below in what is definitely not an exhaustive list perceive cognitive factors (cognition) as the initial mediators of coping-related behaviour.

The fact that an individual has managed a certain performance in the past is an important predictor of the successful use of coping strategies in the future. The theory of self-efficacy (Bandura, 1977), locus of control (Rotter, 1966), the theory of reasoned action (Ajzen, 1991; Ajzen and Fishbein, 1980), attribution theory as well as the theory of perceived control (Thompson, 1981) and powerlessness (Seligman, 1975) see behavioural intention as a key predictor of the pregnant woman's actual behaviour and use of strategies. Powerlessness is described as lack of power (versus control), lack of autonomy and fatalism (Seeman, 1975; Seeman, 1991). Concepts, such as personal control beliefs, locus of control or personal mastery beliefs, reflect the woman's opinion regarding what she can or cannot control or influence (Schultz, Heckhausen and O'Brian, 1994). There is a correlation between control and a "sense of coherence," as a feeling of confidence that the internal and external environment is predictable and that things will work out as expected (Antonovsky, 1979). In contradiction to the personal locus of control, it is not important whether the power to influence results is under our control or not. The feeling of personal control has a significant adaptive effect for the patient. The perceived control is connected with a feeling of subjective comfort, reduced physiological influence of stressors, increased ability to cope with stress, increased activity and lower intensity of pain (Thompson and Spacapan, 1991). A woman needs to feel competent to be able to change her behaviour. A subjective feeling of powerlessness reduces her potential to change the situation, even though she might be able to take active steps. Such low personal control may lead to apathy, and thus reduce positive changes. Catastrophizing is another factor that prevents certain pregnant women from using coping strategies (Sullivan, Rodgers and Kirsch, 2001) or, if they do use them, they still perceive an increased intensity of pain and anxiety and suffer more complications during childbirth (Wuitchik, Hesson and Bakal, 1990). The control of one's own behaviour influences changes in lifestyle in general. Those who prefer to control their own behaviour may make changes while those who do not prefer control may want others to make changes for them (physicians, family, society...) or use another passive approach. An extreme desire to control everything may, however, also have a negative impact on the perceived intensity of pain (Baron Logan and Hoppe, 1993). For example a two-process model of perceived control, distinguish between two types of control: Primary control is an individual's attempt to change the external world or situation so as to accommodate his/her personal needs. Investing time, strength or effort in overcoming obstacles, if any, is a typical example. Secondary control, on the other hand, focuses on the internal world and includes a woman's effort to influence her own motivation, emotions and mental representations (Rothbaum, Weiss and Snyder, 1982). Lazarus and Folkman (1984) explain the difference between primary and secondary control by defining coping that focuses on the problem (primary control) and coping that focuses on emotions (secondary control). Each type of coping relates to different coping strategies. The model shows the understanding of internal processes of behaviour and the differences in using coping strategies under stress (Lefcourt, 1991).

INDIVIDUAL DIMENSION OF COPING STRATEGIES

In coping with labour pain, a woman should use those strategies she personally finds useful in coping with pain or those she has had positive experience with. She can learn such strategies in prenatal courses or even online (Carr, 2004), from the media, friends or family (Henry a Nand, 2004). However, not all women make use of coping strategies in labour or attend prenatal classes; and if they do, not all of the coping strategies are taught in such classes (especially not cognitive ones) (Escott, Spiby, Slade and Fraser, 2004; Escott, Slade, Spiby and Fraser, 2005). Prenatal courses are based on natural childbirth methods (Dick-Read, 1959), prophylaxis (Lamaze, 1956; Bing, 1994) and other methods. They focus on the significance of the childbirth experience, education concerning labour and birth, preparation for parenthood and childcare, bonding with the child, acquiring control over fear from labour and pain and options of analgesia and non-pharmacological approaches. Their effect is to moderate the specific concerns and general anxiety of women having their first baby, thus increasing their confidence to cope with labour and the pain which is perceived as a significant predictor of satisfaction with labour and birth. Although multiparas have had more experience, it is desirable for them to discuss their previous childbirth(s) in the framework of prenatal preparation (Svensson, Barclay and Cooke, 2008).

Thus, the woman will better understand the reasons for e.g., surgical intervention or refusal of pain relief and the probability of problems reoccurring in the forthcoming childbirth. In secundiparas, a talk about emotions during the previous labour is a necessary component of preparation for the next childbirth. After that, the future labour and birth may be planned according to the woman's wishes. However, even providing training in specific coping strategies in prenatal classes does not guarantee that women will actually use those strategies. Of the women who had attended a prenatal course 88% used the breathing technique in coping with pain, 51% used bodywork and only 40% used relaxation (Slade, Escott, Spiby, Henderson and Fraser, 2000). Prenatal courses do not teach cognitive techniques. In coping with labour pain, women prefer the type of coping strategy that they want to use (Rokke and Lall, 1992) or that they have used in the past (Taenzer, 1983). Thus, women can cope with pain in a more effective way if the prenatal course satisfies these individual needs. A woman has an advantage if she has an entire repertoire of strategies to choose from according to the situation, e.g., to specifically cope with labour, pain or anxiety. It is easier for a woman to use well-tried and time-proven coping techniques than it is for her to use newly acquired techniques. The woman's belief about coping with pain during labour plays an important role. It is important for the woman to develop unique coping strategies that will satisfy her preferences and her belief that the selected strategies can help her cope with labour pain (Rokke and al'Absi, 1992). Such a model or prenatal preparation requires the participation of a wide spectrum of experts in prenatal courses, including clinical psychologists, and an individualized approach to the woman's needs.

PLANNING THE USE OF COPING STRATEGIES

The fact that a woman is willing to use coping strategies to manage labour pain, fear of pain and anxiety is important, but not sufficient for her to actually use the strategies. The intention to use various coping strategies is relatively low. Most women come to give birth with a plan to use relaxation breathing only (Slade, Escott, Spiby, Henderson and Fraser, 2000). Preparing a plan of coping strategies may increase the frequency of use of coping strategies during labour. We have already described above that if a woman has previously found any coping strategy useful and effective, she is likely to use such a strategy in the future. Deploying the strategy in a new context of labour pain and labour requires planning which is never easy due to the unpredictability of the childbirth process, the context of pain, environment, reinforcement of positive behaviour, healthcare professionals' and family support and medical or surgical intervention during labour (Escott, Slade and Spiby, 2009). Helping the woman create a plan of coping skills, i.e., when, how and where she can implement certain behaviour, may already be beneficial in the prenatal period. The implementation of coping skills must be equally important for the woman as is the intention. A person's behaviour is intentional and reasoned (Ajzen and Fishbein, 1980). Most of our behaviour patterns are controlled by attitudes rather than social influences (Donald and Cooper, 2001). Therefore, the plan for coping with labour pain should be flexible, in order to accommodate the changing situation during childbirth (Spiby, Slade, Escott, Henderson and Fraser, 2003). The woman should be ready to continue using coping strategies even after disruption or significant change in the direction of the labour, e.g., acute Caesarean section. Doctors may help women use their coping strategies, as well as midwives or partners during labour; they should, however, know the plan, i.e., how and when the woman may wish to use the strategies (Escott, Slade, Spiby and Fraser, 2005). Such women are less likely to require epidural anaesthesia (Copstick, Hayes, Taylor and Morris, 1985). The relationship with the obstetrician (midwife or other healthcare professionals) also has a significant analgesic and anxiolytic effect; for the woman, this is a person who is able to offer empathy and verbal support, evoke trust and create safe conditions for effective support, fear reduction and effective coping with pain.

CONCLUSION

Every woman should be educated on the availability of pharmacological, non-pharmacological and psychologic methods of coping with labour pain. Antenatal preparation should focus on the meaning of pain in labour, psychological and social factors influencing the intensity of pain, and coping with pain and fear of pain. It is further important for a woman to find previously used adaptive coping strategies and learn new strategies (including the often neglected cognitive strategies), maximize the efficiency of selected coping strategies and strengthen her confidence that she can cope with fear, pain and labour even in the context of stress in the delivery room. It is necessary to plan the use of coping strategies. Healthcare professionals and birth partners have an irreplaceable role in supporting women in actually using the selected unique coping strategies in labour. They should be knowledgeable of psychological coping techniques in order to encourage women to use them.

Such an approach requires a multidisciplinary team, from obstetricians, anaesthesiologists, clinical psychologists and psychotherapists to nurses and midwives and other healthcare professionals, not only in labour but also during prenatal preparation and care.

In: The Psychological Context of Labour Pain   ISBN: 978-1-63483-825-2
Editors: J. Raudenská and A. Javůrková © 2016 Nova Science Publishers, Inc.

Chapter 4

FEAR AND LABOUR PAIN

Jaroslava Raudenská, Antonella Paladini
and Alena Javůrková

ABSTRACT

The joy from the birth of a new life would not exist without the
experience of pain, fear and potential danger. A woman may subjectively
perceive labour pain as part of the birth, as a positive power, or as
inevitable suffering; this has to do with her personal story and socio-
cultural specifics. The first part of this chapter focuses on the relationship
between the following concepts as frequently used in communication
between pregnant women and healthcare professionals: pain, suffering,
loss and support. The chapter further describes anxiety and fear of labour
pain and their treatment. Coping with the fear of labour pain should be
facilitated by a multidisciplinary team able to offer a wide variety of
pharmacological and non-pharmacological pain relief methods and
specific forms of psychotherapy.

Keywords: fear, anxiety, pregnancy, labour and birth, support, psychotherapy,
cognitive-behavioural therapy

INTRODUCTION

In light ofthe fast changes in the Western society, the significance of motherhood has, over the last years, been pushed aside in favour of work and career. The birth of a child requires mastering new skills and accepting new responsibilities (Ruble, Brooks-Gunn, Fleming, Fitzmaurice, Stang or and Deutsch, 1990). The transition to parenthood is a developmental process leading to maturity – at the end of this process both the woman and the man reach a permanent change. Adolescent women, older primiparas and women who do not have a partner or psychosocial support are more vulnerable in the transition to parenthood. During the *first trimester*, the woman's original identity is threatened; unconscious anxiety, sadness over the loss of her own childhood and fear of regression are quite common. During the *second trimester*, the woman adapts to the approaching motherhood and perceives the child as an independent being. Unconscious anxiety subsides to be replaced by concerns about the child's welfare. The *third trimester* reflects active preparation for labour, the child and the new life situation. Emotional and social withdrawal together with lower interest in external stimuli help the woman concentrate on labour and birth and labour pain. By birth, the woman loses her symbiotic connection with the child which may also cause certain anxiety. An early relationship between the mother and the child and bonding (Bowlby, 1969) are key for the child's emotional wellbeing and optimum development; such a connection is already developing during pregnancy (Hipwell, Goossens, Melhuish and Kumar, 2000). The birth of a child to the family is one of the most significant interpersonal changes.

PAIN AND SUFFERING

A woman may subjectively perceive labour pain as part of birth, a positive power, a major test of her femininity and personal competence and the first step to motherhood, or as inevitable and irrational suffering and danger; this has to do with her personal story and socio-cultural specifics. In order to understand fear of labour pain, it is important to understand the terms pain and suffering. Pain and suffering are sometimes used as synonyms, and although they are closely related, each of them has a different meaning. Pain relates to a conscious experience of somatic, emotional or spiritual discomfort that is outside the individual's control. Suffering exceeds the conscious experience of discomfort and means the pain's impact on the woman's attitude to and cognitive processing of pain, i.e., acceptance, indifference or rejection connected with pain (Price, 2002).

Suffering in general can be characterised as a perceived threat that may affect the body or the psychosocial self, or both, as a complex adverse emotional experience, or as a permanent psychological condition (Chapman and Gavrin, 1993). The above definition of suffering, however, does not explain the exhilaration of people seeking adventure in dangerous situations. In reaction to danger, an individual may experience excitement and exhilaration rather than suffering, if the individual trusts himself/herself to be able to effectively cope with the challenge. Powerlessness and suffering, on the other hand, are experienced if the individual facing danger is unable to cope with it. A situation in which a woman in labour subjectively feels that she is unable to cope with labour pain may help us understand why such procedures as, for instance, the woman's preparation for birth, empathy, support from healthcare professionals, and non-pharmacological strategies of coping with pain may enhance a woman's ability to cope with labour pain, without the necessity of reducing the sensory component of the intensity of pain. Non-pharmacological strategies can reduce the woman's feeling of powerlessness and may improve the level of (or even prevent) suffering.

In order to understand the experience of suffering, we need to explore the concept of loss (from the somatic, psychological, and social perspective). The woman may feel potential loss resulting from the loss of self, loss of familiar environment, threat to her somatic integrity during labour and birth, or concern about her own death or the death of the child. All this may be expressed as fear of labour and labour pain. Women across cultures who fear pain and labour are particularly worried about the health of their child and loss of control and personal integrity during labour, and fear somatic injury and pain (Lowe, 2000).

Pain and suffering may sometimes appear separately. If the woman understands the origin of her pain (cervical dilation and the descending foetus), she perceives labour as highly positive (pain for her is a "good" sign of progress leading to a goal) and understands the related pain as an experience that is not life threatening and that she can cope with; she may experience pain of high intensity, but not suffering. This is the main reason why certain women defend labour without analgesia, although the pain experienced in labour is of a high intensity. For these women, even a high intensity of pain brings a significant feeling of harmony and joy that may coexist with and be independent of the experience of labour and labour pain.

Labour and the birth of a new life become a life experience that can be coped with and can help the woman experience success and improve her own self-confidence. A positive experience and positive emotions may thus be independent of the intensity of pain during labour.

ANXIETY AND FEAR

About 20% of all pregnancies in economically developed countries are complicated because of anxiety during pregnancy, and fear of pain, suffering and labour (Saisto, Salmela-Aro, Nurmi and Halmesmäki, 2001a). Anxiety and fear related to pregnancy, labour and labour pain are considered in the context of anxiety disorders which may include generalized anxiety disorder, health anxiety, specific phobias (algophobia, tocophobia), post-traumatic stress disorder(PTSD), or acute stress reaction.

We can generally identify three dimensions of birth-related anxiety: pregnancy, labour and birth, and the postnatal period. Prenatal anxiety and the influence of prenatal anxiety on pregnancy and coping with pain and labour are explored using questionnaires (see in appendix 1) designed to measure not just general anxiety, but also its specific content. Anxiety in pregnancy is constant and does not decrease until the second trimester, rising again in the third trimester. Anxiety may express itself as various somatic complaints, e.g., stomach pain, headaches or nausea, and may result in frequent visits to the gynaecologist or maternity hospital. Individual personality traits linked to anxiety influence how the woman anticipates and experiences various events in her life, including pregnancy, labour and pain. Anxiety in pregnancy and during labour may be co-created by conflicts in pregnancy, social and financial insecurity, or insufficient information (Saisto, Salmela-Aro, Nurmi and Halmesmäki, 2001a). There is a correlation between anxiety, fear, high levels of stress during pregnancy, adverse perinatal results and increased soreness in labour.

Fear of labour pain is linked to a general fear of pain in other situations. It may involve primary fear typical in primiparas and be connected with the pre morbid psychopathology of anxiety disorders, or it may involve secondary fear resulting from previous negative experiences (with insufficient pain relief during previous birth, disappointment with previous vaginal labour, etc.). The background of fear of labour may be psychological (mental problems prior to pregnancy, personality disorders, previous traumatic events or fear of future parenthood, low self-confidence and self-esteem, major everyday life stressors) or social (lack of social support, economic insecurity, the mother's low age, education or socioeconomic status, lack of knowledge, and lack of prenatal preparation).

Fear of labour pain is reported by one half of all pregnant women. 6-10% of women suffer irrational fear of pain (Geissbuehler and Eberhard, 2002). These patients do not change their evaluation of pain even after opiate analgesia and are better able to cope with pain after reducing anxiety (Janssen and Arntz, 2001). Irrational and inadequate fear (algophobia, i.e., a specific type of phobia) leads to stronger reactions to painful signals (hyper vigilance) that are evaluated as dangerous and, if possible, avoided (Raudenska, Javurkova and Kozak, 2013; Vlaeyen, Morley, Linton, Boersma and De Jong, 2012). Behaviour aimed at the avoidance of pain is connected with anxiety. Anxious women more frequently require epidural analgesia and C-section and report a higher intensity of pain and fear of pain, and worse cooperation with healthcare personnel during labour (Rouhe, Salmela-Aro, Halmesmäki and Saisto, 2009). Generalized anxiety applies to pregnancy, labour and birth, the result of the birth process, consequences for the woman, and other worries. Thanks to the release of endogenous opioids initiated by anxiety during pregnancy and labour, pain is better tolerated. Increased anxiety during labour, on the other hand, is related to increased pain intensity (Waldenström, Hildingsson and Ryding, 2006). The increased secretion of catecholamine may increase nociception from the pelvis and strengthen the perception of nociceptive stimuli on the cortical level (Lowe, 1996), thus extending the first stage of labour (Alehagen, Wijma, K. and Wijma, B., 2006). One third of the partners of women who showed fear of labour and labour pain also reported fear; one fifth of these men requested a Caesarean section for their female partner (Sjögren and Thomassen, 1997).

Fear of labour pain is closely related to fear of inability to give birth (tocophobia); a woman may fear that she will do something wrong and, due to her incompetent behaviour during labour, she may harm the child or herself (Szeverenyi, Poka, Hetey and Torok, 1998). This is often accompanied by fear of losing self-control or contact with reality and feelings of hopelessness and helplessness. The above concerns may result either from a traumatic event in childhood (e.g., abuse or abandonment) or previous experiences of rejection (e.g., during previous interaction with healthcare). This may further lead to alack of self-confidence in contact with the delivery room personnel, a deepening of feelings of despair and helplessness, and lower compliance.

Birth can be traumatic. Medical problems can be frightening. Unbearable labour pain and unexpected complications (e.g., in the form of acute Caesarean section, the near death of a mother or baby, heavy bleeding or premature birth) are considered possible causes of Posttraumatic Stress Disorder (PTSD). Emotional difficulties in coping with the pain of childbirth can also cause psychological trauma. Childbirth related PTSD can be caused even by a normal birth. Even if others perceive the birth as normal, if the mother perceives it as traumatic, it was traumatic. PTSD is an extended reaction to an experience that involved danger of death or severe harm to oneself or a close person. The disorder is characterised by anxiety and recurring flashbacks of the event, effort to avoid similar situations, flattened emotional response and sleep disorders. Factors contributing to predisposition to PTSD in pregnant women include previous mental disorders or negative experience as patients, first delivery, failure to cope with pain, feelings of insecurity or exposure to risk during labour, bad relationships with a partner, and difficulty with accepting pregnancy and the transition to parenthood (Ryding, Wijma, B. and Wijma, K., 1997).

TREATMENT

Women who fear labour and labour pain may be treated by health professionals from various fields.

Preparation for labour facilitated by midwifery personnel involves education on labour, pain and the range of pharmacological and non-pharmacological methods of coping with pain available at the given facility, with the aim of controlling the fear of labour and labour pain. In the case of secondary fear of labour, a dialogue between the obstetrician and the woman about her previous labour may help resolve any misunderstanding (Graham, Hundley, McCheyne, Hall, Gurney and Milne, 1999). If the woman understands the reasons for e.g., a surgical intervention and its consequences, the refusal of a certain type of pain relief, or the probability of recurrence of problems in the forthcoming labour, she will be able to see the difference between the previous situation and the current situation. Planning both the medication and non-pharmacological methods of coping with pain is very important. Primiparas with a fear of labour should be guaranteed that there are pain relief options to help them concentrate on aspects other than pain.

Support provided by a healthcare professional in the form of "being there with and for the woman in labour" means that the woman can express her needs, not only physical, but also emotional and spiritual. This gives the woman in labour a feeling of relief, security, physical and mental well being, hope and expectation, including the satisfaction of her somatic and psychological needs, and positive expectations. This explains why women who receive comfort, safety, information and support for their coping skills in the form of encouragement, emotional support and a humane approach are able not to only cope with pain, but even experience their own power during labour (Lundgren and Dahlberg, 1998). Women who describe their experience with labour pain often stress the paradox between pain and support. Some women for instance, cannot describe the pain, deny it or use contradictive statements ("It was hell ... nobody helped me ... I felt a little pain ... anyway, I had to somehow cope with it on my own ...").

Psychotherapy. Cognitive Behavioural Therapy (CBT) techniques offered by a clinical psychologist with accredited training are effective in coping with fear of pain and stress and in increasing self-confidence. CBT is based on the assumption that the woman does not react primarily to direct external stimuli of her environment, but to her cognitive representation of the environment. The learning process is based on the stimulus-organism-response-consequence formula. Cognitive processes function as a mediator between stimulus and behaviour. It is not only the stimulus (e.g., abdominal contractions) that produces a particular behaviour (flight, escape, scream), but the meaning the woman has assigned to the stimulus (e.g., "something is wrong," "I am going to die," "The child is dying," etc.) that produces tension and increased pain. (At the same time CBT does not neglect the physiological pain mechanisms and the pain perception). Consequences reinforce or weaken certain behaviour based on the meaning assigned to the consequences by the woman. Women with increased anxiety or fear of pain and labour are indicated for individual or group therapy in pregnancy. The aim of psychotherapy is to teach the patient how to see a problem from a different perspective (self-reflection) and change the procedures connected with the target problem. Constructive thinking and coping skills already reduce anxiety and fear in pregnancy, both directly and indirectly. CBT techniques such as education, cognitive restructuring, self-instruction, in-imagination exposure, modeling, role playing, and problem solving are commonly used in the prenatal period to reduce anxiety and fear of labour pain. Other techniques work to reduce anxiety and fear during labour: attention distraction, hypnosis, biofeedback, relaxation, guided imagination, progressive muscle relaxation, meditation and deep breathing (Raudenska, Amlerova and Javurkova, 2014).

Studies investigating the results of psychotherapy in women with fear of labour pain are rare (Saisto and Halmesmäki, 2003). The effects of treating anxiety and fear of labour pain could be evaluated by the decrease of perceived stress and better compliance during pregnancy, but also by the number of withdrawn requests for "CS on demand" (see more details in Chapter 5).

CONCLUSION

In order to understand labour pain, we need to understand the relationship between life and death, pain and giving new life, fear, hope, and joy. The context of labour and birth, pain, suffering, support and stress allows certain women to experience labour as a significant event in their lives even though it is painful and uncomfortable. Some women are scared of labour pain and a few try to avoid pain at any cost, as their fear is irrational and inadequate. All women should therefore be educated on the availability of pharmacological, non-pharmacological and psychotherapeutical pain relief methods. Prevention of fear of pain and coping with fear assume the cooperation of obstetricians, anaesthesiologists, clinical psychologists and other healthcare professionals. Psychotherapy may help the woman learn new coping strategies and build up her own self-confidence to cope with fear, pain and labour. Trust, assurance, safety, support and encouragement provided by healthcare personnel and birth partners in the delivery room have a significant analgesic and anxiolytic effect and contribute to fear reduction and effective coping. These facts may contribute to coping with fear of labour pain in clinical practice, but also to the area of research and education of healthcare professionals, women in labour and the general public.

APPENDIX 1. THE EXAMPLES OF QUESTIONNAIRES DESIGNED TO MEASURE GENERAL ANXIETY AND ALSO ITS SPECIFIC CONTENT

Spielberger's state-trait anxiety inventory (STAI)
Beck Anxiety Inventory (BAI)
Perinatal Anxiety Screening Scale (PASS)
Pregnancy-Related Anxiety Questionnaire
Cambridge Worry Scale
Prenatal Distress Questionnaire
Positive and Negative Affect Schedule
Prenatal Self-Evaluation Questionnaire

In: The Psychological Context of Labour Pain   ISBN: 978-1-63483-825-2
Editors: J. Raudenská and A. Javůrková © 2016 Nova Science Publishers, Inc.

Chapter 5

CAESAREAN SECTION ON MATERNAL REQUEST

Jaroslava Raudenská and Alena Javůrková

ABSTRACT

The initial part of Chapter Five summarises the incidence of, indications for, and certain social, cultural, economic and psychological reasons for the growing number of Caesarean sections. Over the last decade, a woman's right to choose the method of birth and Caesarean section "on demand" without medical indication have become the topics of heated debate. This chapter discusses the reasons for caesarean section on maternal request, the advantages and disadvantages of caesarean delivery without medical indication, the influence of the obstetrician and female patient's cognitive factors on the method of childbirth, ethical aspects with anemphasis on partnership with the obstetrician and possible methods of supporting the women concerned. The chapter concludes that prenatal care should start as early as possible, preferably during pregnancy, and should involve a multidisciplinary team to overcome the causes of fear of labour pain and vaginal birth.

Keywords: fear of labour, labour pain and delivery, ethical aspects, partnership, support

INTRODUCTION

Over the last fifty years, the hospital has become the standard place for the delivery of babies. Over the same period, we have observed an increasing number of caesarean deliveries. Before World War II, the proportion of Caesarean sections (CSs) was less than 1% of all deliveries. In 1970, CSs in most economically developed countries accounted for 5% of all deliveries, in the 1980s for 10% and after 1985 for 15-20%. In e.g., Italy or Tai-wan, the number of CSs increased to 60%. According to WHO, major increases in CS rates, i.e., by 70%, have been recorded in Latin America; about 40% of all babies here are born by caesarean section. In large city hospitals in Brazil, as many as 80% of all babies are born by CS (Lauer, Betrán, Merialdi and Wojdyla, 2010). Giving birth by CS is "in." For example, 31% of all deliveries in the USA were concluded with a CS in 2006 (Rossi and D'Addario, 2008) and in 2009 the number increased to 32.9% (Martin, Hamilton, Ventura, Osterman, Wilson and Mathews, 2012). In Sweden on the other hand, the CS rate is only 17% (Wiklund, Andolf, Lilja and Hildingsson, 2012). According to WHO, the optimal CS rate is 10-15% of all deliveries. Increasing the rate does not help reduce perinatal mortality and morbidity, even in the most advanced perinatology centres (Wagner, 1994; WHO, 2015).

REASONS FOR GROWING CAESAREAN SECTION RATES

Pregnancy and birth are increasingly seen as something unnatural, a disease that needs to be treated, and the Caesarean section is a safe operation, the safety of which is comparable to that of vaginal delivery. The extensive rise in CS rates, however, appears to be particularly due to socio-economic and psychological reasons (Kennare, 2003). In addition, the relationship between the obstetrician and the woman and the status of obstetricians and that of pregnant women are constantly changing in relation to the legal and ethical background.

Most women in economically developed countries deliver their babies in hospitals, and more deliveries, particularly in private hospitals (Easter, 2015), lead to more Caesarean sections. The average age of first-time mothers has also increased and so has the risk of possible complications which may lead to a decision to perform a caesarean delivery. Certain obstetricians may prefer to plan a CS in older women in order to feel that they have better control over the birth process. The increased use of epidural anaesthesia in vaginal childbirth is another trend; the woman may avoid feeling any pain whatsoever (Michales, 2012). The increasing number of cases of induced labour may also contribute to increased CS rates, as may higher rates of multiple pregnancies due to assisted reproduction and the fact that women who have had one CS are more likely to have another (Verdult, 2009). Physicians' attempts to protect themselves is another reason for the performance of Caesarean sections; in case of complications, they can say they did their best to save both the mother and the child. A "prudent obstetrician" may prefer to conclude a labour with surgery. Consequently, we see higher CS rates among celebrities, female doctors and obstetricians' partners (Al-Mufti, McCarthy and Fisk, 1996). In interviews conducted with obstetricians, up to one half of the respondents believed that it was the media and women's requests that were behind increasing CS rates (Usha Kiran and Jayawickrama, 2002). Women are used to making their own choices. The paternalistic model of the relationship between the obstetrician and the female patient is slowly changing in favour of a cooperative pattern of relationships; under the latter, the obstetrician should be equipped with certain communication and supportive psychotherapy skills. Finally, the reasons for increased CS rates may include a general lack of interest in the psychological, sociological and cultural aspects of pregnancy and coping with labour and labour pain among of some healthcare professionals (Odent, 2004).

PREVALENCE OF CAESAREAN SECTIONS ON MATERNAL REQUEST

Over the last decade, voices have been raised for the woman's right to plan parenthood, terminate unwanted pregnancies, discuss prenatal diagnostics and choose her obstetrician, home labour, her position during labour, and the method of labour (Quadros, 2000), as well as any analgesia to be applied (Michaels, 2012). Requests to perform a Caesarean section "on demand" probably originated in Brasil (Finger, 2003). It is very difficult to determine their prevalence as there may be other indications for CSs. In Great Britain, caesarean deliveries at the mother's request accounted for 1-2% of all deliveries, 7-14% of all CS deliveries and up to 30% of all non-acute CSs with the woman's significant involvement in the decision to perform a CS (Nama and Wilcock, 2011). In Australia, 17% of all optional CSs are caesarean deliveries on maternal request (CDMR), i.e., about 3% of all deliveries (D´Souza and Arulkumaran, 2013). In Sweden, CDMR account for about 8% of all CSs that constitute 17% of all deliveries (Wiklund, Andolf, Lilja and Hildingsson, 2012). In the USA, about 2.5% of all deliveries are estimated to be CDMR (2006). In Italy, a woman's right to choose the method of childbirth has recently been enacted. In the first year after the law was ratified, 4% of all CSs were CDMR (Tranquilli and Garzetti, 1997). One in every five Italian women expressed a preference for CS (Torloni, Betrán, Montilla, Scolaro et al., 2013). In southeast China, this type of delivery is chosen by up to 20% of women (Zhang, Liu, Meikle, Zheng, Sun and Li, 2008).

REASONS FOR CAESAREAN DELIVERIES ON MATERNAL REQUEST

A woman's motives for choosing a caesarean delivery may include fear of the birth process, fear of the consequences of vaginal delivery, bad experiences with childbirth, and emotional and social problems (Andersson, Sundström-Poromaa, Bixo et al., 2003; Hall and Bewley, 1999; Nama and Wilcock, 2011).

Fear of the Birth Process

Certain woman may perceive natural birth as a high-risk and uncontrollable process; in comparison, CS has a script and provides a certain level of certainty. Although CS causes exhaustion, longer recovery periods and postoperative pain, a woman's attempt to deliver a child by CS on request may be driven by an exaggerated fear of labour pain during vaginal delivery. However, CS may disturb bonding, care of the baby and breast feeding. Women who requested CS had, compared to a control group of women who opted for vaginal delivery, the following thoughts: they were not in good health, wanted only one child, and were afraid of having little control over their labour. After the planned CS, women from the group described better experiences with childbirth than the women after vaginal delivery. Unfortunately, compared to the women who had had vaginal delivery, they breastfed their babies for less than three months (Wiklund, Edman and Andolf, 2007).

Fear of Consequences of Vaginal Delivery

Certain women are driven to request CS by fear of damage to the foetus during the labour process, changes in the anatomy of the birth canal, incontinence, and negative consequences for their sex life. Some women wish to start sexual activity early after birth or influence the child's date of birth. Long-term failed artificial insemination may also influence requests for CS. Finally, the higher a woman's socioeconomic status, the more often she requests CDMR (Barley, Aylin, Bottle and Jarman,2004).

Experience with Labour

Requests for CDMR are affected by women's experiences with labour. In primiparas, the most frequent reasons include fear of pain, fear of labour and a desire to control the birth and the date of birth. In multiparas, reasons include previous complicated vaginal delivery (tearing, uterine prolapse or urinary or faecal incontinence) (Wiklund, Andolf, Lilja and Hildingsson,2012) and inappropriate pain relief. Women who have already had an acute CS often wish to have the same procedure during their next childbirth (Hildingsson, Rĺdestad, Rubertsson and Waldenström, 2002).

Emotional and Social Issues

Psychosis. Women suffering from psychotic disorders and who are stabilized may go for a vaginal delivery after psychological preparation and education. The decision should be made on the basis of communication with the woman and the opinion of a multidisciplinary team including a psychiatrist and a psychotherapist.

Pre-and post-traumatic stress disorder. Women requesting a CS have a bigger fear of labour and pain, lower socialization scores, higher anxiety and more symptoms of depression. These may be risk factors for pre- and post-traumatic stress disorders (PTSD). About 2% of women suffer from PTSD after childbirth (Ayers, Eagle and Waring, 2006; Söderquist, Wijma and Thorbert et al., 2009), which may have a significant impact on their attitude to subsequent pregnancies.

Sexual abuse. Women who are victims of abuse, sexual abuse or other forms of violence or women with severe traumatic experiences (wars, catastrophes) may request a CS. They often think that during a vaginal delivery they would be helpless, with no control over the situation and that the experience could bring up their negative memories (Burian, 1995). These should include careful follow-up of traumatized women to check for memory distortions over time, as well as the use of sophisticated techniques, such as brain imaging, to gain further understanding about the ways the central nervous system processes traumatic memories. There clearly is a need for further studies of dissociative processes and their relationship to the development and maintenance of PTSD (Van der Kolk and Fisler, 1995).

Fear of labour and pain. About 6–20% of women suffer from to cophobia, i.e., an irrational fear of labour (National Collaborating Centre for Women's and Children's Health, 2004) which is one of the major causes of CDMR. Women with fear of labour often consider vaginal delivery risky and generally prefer medical and surgical intervention (Greer, Lazenbatt and Dunne, 2014). They are afraid of damage to the pelvic floor, injury to or death of the child, and feelings of loneliness during labour. Womenwho experience a strong fear of labour during pregnancy perceive labour pain more intensively than women who do not experience fear during pregnancy (Haines, Rubertsson, Pallant and Hildingsson, 2012). Fear of labour pain and labour was the motive for 7-22% of all non-acute CSs in Sweden and Great Britain (MacKenzie, 1999), for example.

Obstetricians' motives for choosing CS for their own childbirth. Obstetricians tend to choose caesarean delivery rather than vaginal delivery in their or their partner's childbirth, which is particularly driven by their fear of perineal trauma or sexual dysfunction and concerns about the child's health (Finsen, Storeheier and Aasland, 2008). While nearly all midwives opt for vaginal delivery, obstetricians prefer CSs for both themselves and their families (Dickson and Willett, 1999). Physicians frequently attend complicated childbirths and, as a result, their fear of their or their partner's labour may increase (Aslam, Gilmour and Fawdry, 2003).

The relationship between a woman and her obstetrician has a significant impact on the woman's request for CS. Studies from Brazil and Chile show that CS rates increaseas a result of women's requests (Potter, Berquó, Perpétuo, Leal, Hopkins and Souza et al., 2001; Potter and Hopkins 2002), but mainly due to the relationship between the woman and her obstetrician (Nama and Wilcock 2011).

IMPACT OF THE PHYSICIAN'S ATTITUDE ON THE METHOD OF CHILDBIRTH AND BIRTH MANAGEMENT

The physician's behaviour, i.e., the proposed method of childbirth, and the female patient's subsequent decision is influenced by cognitive factors (beliefs, ideas, opinions, evaluations) (Broome, 1989). A physician's approach may vary with each patient, which can hardly be explained by the physician's professional knowledge only. A physician's individual model of health and disease and personal opinion on what he/she would do in the patient´s position are of a particular relevance. A patient's final decision is based on three different types of the physician's authority: 1. Generally accepted authority; this results from the physician's professional commitment to mediate advice for the patient while the effect depends on the patient's acceptance, 2. Professional authority; the doctor is the one with superior medical education, 3. Informative authority; this type depends on the reliability and convincingness of the information provided to the patient by the doctor.

While advising the patient on the methods of delivery and coping with pain, the medical doctor makes use of his/her professional knowledge as well as his/her personal opinion. The extent to which a patient is willing to accept the doctor's advice may depend on her comprehension of the information, ability to memorize it, and her general satisfaction with the consultation. Advice provided by an obstetrician has a certain "frame." This means the context and situation of the case (Ley, 1985). For example, medical students recommended surgery to their patients if they had information that surgery was the only possible solution (i.e., positive frame) in contrast to a negative frame (Miller, Fagley and Casella, 2009). In addition to the obstetrician's selected procedure, negative or positive framing also affects the patient's selection of the method of childbirth and pain relief. The patient's opinion is rarely identical with or even similar to that of the doctor. Their opinions on the method and place of childbirth, compliance with the principles of work during pregnancy etc., may differ dramatically. The influence of the medical doctor's cognitive factors on the patient's decision regarding childbirth is not a direct one, but one that relates to other factors in the biopsychosocial model of health and disease.

ETHICAL ASPECTS AND CMDR

Medical ethics is a type of moral philosophy, i.e., a moral commitment governing the practice of medicine, including obstetrics. In medical ethics, a commitment is a set of rights and obligations and ethics is about rights, errors, good and evil. Obstetrics is governed by ethics; not the other way round. Medical ethics has its source in religion and philosophy and may drive doctors to varying courses of action. Ethics also relates to the obstetrician's nature and personality as shaped by virtues. An obstetrician becomes an expert through his/her virtues, honour and integrity rather than by completing studies at a medical faculty or specializing in obstetrics. Like all medical doctors, obstetricians observe four key ethical principles: 1. Non-male ficence (avoiding harm to the patient); 2. Beneficence (acting in the best interest of the patient); 3. Autonomy (including respect for the patient's values as expressed through her informed consent and participation in treatment); 4. Justice. For example, pain relief during labour is a classic example of the application of the principles of doing no harm to the patient and respecting the best interests of the patient, towards beneficence (Beauchamp and Childress, 2001). The right to choose CS without medical indication is a burning question in view of the ethical principle of doing no harm to the woman, i.e., avoiding any risks and any damage, to beneficence. Failure to grant are quest for CS on demand may be considered a failure to meet the ethical principle of autonomy. If, however, the patient's autonomy is the only concept respected, the doctor's judgement is devalued. Therefore, the woman's unique wishes must be considered in the socio-cultural context (Devendra and Arulkumaran, 2003). Ensuring the quality of information available to women requesting a Caesarean section and determining whether a woman is considered informed, are other ethical dilemmas, as is the question of whether it is the woman who requests a CS or the obstetrician who gives her the choice and whether and how, in such cases, fear of labour pain is diagnosed and treatment is offered. Another ethical dilemma is that the care of pregnant women under a state-subsidised healthcare system has certain limits and CDMR may have a negative impact on other people's right to access medical care. Resources from society should be allocated to healthcare wisely and evidence-based treatment with clear health benefits should be supported (Schenker and Cain, 1999). On the other hand, helping a woman who is giving birth to a baby is an interest that supersedes the interests of others. Decisions regarding the execution of CDMR are then affected by the principle of justice.

DOCTOR-PATIENT PARTNERSHIP

Cooperation between the obstetrician and the patient increases compliance in the process of childbirth and in the selection of analgesia. Extreme forms of the relationship and of the patient's share in decision making include the doctor's monopoly (a paternalistic model) or decisions made solely by the patient (an informed choice). Between these two extremes, there are joint decisions (a cooperative model) (Koerfer, Albus and Obliers, et al., 2008). The paternalistic, service-oriented and cooperative models are the most frequent models of relationship between a patient and physician; various versions of the models are possible. In practice, the models may blend and extreme versions only exist in theory. Under the paternalistic model, the patient has the right to refuse, but not to request treatment that is considered risky or not medically justified. The doctor's role is directive; the doctor requires the patient's obedience and has a therapeutic "privilege." For a patient who wants a CS, this model means that the doctor will not discuss her wishes with her. Under the informative model, the patient is expected to have sufficient medical knowledge to make the right decision. The negotiation model falls between the paternalistic and the informative models. The doctor exchanges information with the patient, providing her with sufficient empathy and independence of decision while guiding her towards the optimum decision. Highly educated women typically want to make their own choices regarding treatment and to make their own decisions; this, however, does not apply in general (Vick and Scott, 1998). A contractual model is the opposite of the paternalistic model. The patient understands the doctor as a service; the doctor is an "expert" but the amount of information and treatment is decided by the patient herself. Under the cooperative model, the doctor helps the patient determine a treatment plan in compliance with her values and wishes using negotiation and ending with a joint decision and joint responsibility for treatment. The doctor is interested in the patient's feelings and mood, psychosocial problems or cultural specifics. This model presumes a deeper use of psychological approach, the doctor's communication skills and supportive psychotherapy. In case of a request for CS, ethical principles can be met by a cooperative relationship between the obstetrician and the patient, repeated consultations with a single doctor (or team), multidisciplinary care, and healthcare provided to the woman in the prenatal period.

Pros and Cons of CDMR

The reasons for a particular woman to request CS without medical indication may vary. The reasons for surgical delivery should be assessed with sufficiency. The important thing is that the woman gives a reason that maybe subject to multidisciplinary consultation. Specific guidelines should be adopted for such requests accordingly (Wiklund, Andolf, Lilja and Hildingsson, 2012).

Cons

CDMR adversaries point out the higher risks involved in surgery (the risk of maternal death is increased up to 16-fold) and the stagnation of perinatological indicators as a result of the growing number of CSs. They desire strict observance of the medical indications for surgical delivery. In their opinion, the method is expensive and draws on healthcare resources that may be needed elsewhere. A woman's request for CS should only be granted if medical indications exist (Easter, 2015). As already described in the section on increasing CS rates, the increasing age of pregnant women is one indicator. *According to CDMR adversaries, however, a woman's age should not automatically be grounds for granting the request.* Some women insist on their request even though they have attended multidisciplinary consultations in perinatal centres. The adversaries do not consider this to be a reason for granting a request without medical indication if the woman has been informed about the advantages of a vaginal delivery and is able to give vaginal birth. Feelings of inadequacy, guilt, and failure in not completing a natural process may affect bonding between mother and infant, particularly if the operation was conducted under general anaesthetic.

Pros

CDMR fans argue that both economic reasons and clinical data against such requests are inconclusive. This means that a woman's request would be in conflict with the doctor's decision, contradicting the principle of justice. From the point of view of the ethical principle of autonomy, the woman's wish is of utmost importance and should not be rejected (Gee, 2015). Refusal of a woman's request for CDMR is a sign of a strictly paternalistic relationship between the obstetrician and the patient and allows the doctor to decide without discussing the woman's wishes or giving her a chance to speak up. Treating a woman as a passive being is unethical. The woman's wishes should always be the subject of communication between the obstetrician and the patient, as described in the "Doctor-Patient Partnership" section of this Chapter. In general, medicine has an inclination to vaginal delivery; certain obstetricians see women who request CS without medical indication as difficult and the requested method of childbirth as inappropriate. If the woman has a reason for such a request, e.g., fear of labour, pain, or any other type of birth-related fear, she should be referred to a psychotherapist who is a member of the perinatal centre team.

In deciding whether to approve a CDMR, an obstetrician needs to consider all short and long-term health consequences for both the woman and the child; the risk of CS should also be considered against the risk of not granting the request. Some women who refuse spontaneous delivery but are not granted their request for CS may enforce a CS during labour. This is much more dangerous than a planned CS (Wiklund, Andolf, Lilja and Hildingsson,2012). If a patient has been through psychotherapy and other consultations and still insists on her request, it should be granted. Specific guidelines should be implemented for those women who could benefit from CDMR (D´Souza and Arulkumaran, 2013).

Healthcare professionals do not share the same opinion on women's requests for CS. Although some liberal obstetricians support women's autonomy and agree with granting requests for CS without medical indication, the reasons for such requests should always be investigated and identified as they typically involve fear and other psychosocial disorders.

RECOMMENDATION AND SUPPORT

Women have to be first of all educated about pros and cons of vaginal delivery. One of the benefits of having a vaginal birth is that it has a shorter hospital stay and recovery time compared with a C-section. Women who undergo vaginal births avoid major surgery and its associated risks (severe bleeding, scarring, infections, reactions to an aesthesia and more longer-lasting pain) and could hold the baby and begin breastfeeding sooner after delivering, what speeding up the bonding process. During a vaginal delivery it makes babies less likely to suffer breathing problems at birth. Vaginally birth also may boost infant´s immune systems and protect intestinal tracts. On the other hand the vaginal delivery can be stressful, long. Some deliveries are short while others take hours depending on each case. A very small percentage of babies may experience injury during vaginal birth. Three key strategies supports the normalization of birth: 1. an "ethos" of normality of vaginal birth; 2. "working" the evidence; and 3. "trusting" women to make informed choices best for them (Kennedy, Grant, Walton, Shaw-Battista and Sandall, 2010).

If a woman still requests CS, all specific risk factors should be considered, e.g., her age, body mass index, further plans concerning maternity, emotional disorders, personal values and the social and cultural context. It is very important to obtain the woman´s medical, pharmacological, psychological and social history. Women should receive information on the advantages, disadvantages, and consequences, both short-term and long-term, of a CS for both the woman and the baby. Finding the woman's reasons for her request is always better than intimidating her by telling her about the risks. Depending on her reasons, the woman should have consultations with other members of the team (psychiatrist, psychologist, psychotherapist, midwife, social worker or physiotherapist). Clinics with multidisciplinary teams report the highest rates of satisfaction with labour and birth among women (Waldenström, Hildingsson and Ryding, 2006).

Integrated multidisciplinary health care provided to a woman during pregnancy and prior to and during childbirth may prevent her request for CS altogether. Women who experience fear of pain, labour, the consequences of vaginal birth or emotional and social difficulties *early in pregnancy* should be diagnosed and offered a therapy (Wiklund, Edman, Ryding and Andolf, 2008). The responsability have the gynaecologists while taking care of the pregnancy. Women who have suffered from severe stress reactions due to traumatic childbirth experiences and insufficient pain relief should be offered psychotherapy and crisis intervention. Various emotional problems, particularly fear and the nature of that fear, of a woman requesting CS prior to delivery should be adequately explored in order to offer the woman relief. If the reason for her request for CS is fear of labour and labour pain, she should have consultations with an anaesthesiologist, psychotherapist, psychiatrist, obstetrician and midwife. Vaginal deliveries in women with irrational fear of labour pain and childbirth who had been treated and then withdrew their request after treatment were successful, but with higher rates of induced labour, oxytocin use and epidural analgesia (Sjögren and Thomassen, 1997). About 50% to 86% of women requesting CS (Ryding, 1993) choose vaginal delivery after regular psychotherapy (Nerum, Halvorsen, Sorlie and Oian,2006);their satisfaction with labour is higher than that in women who had no fear of labour and pain. However, up to one third of women with fear of labour and labour pain refused the support offered (Wiklund, Edman, Larsson and Andolf, 2009). If a woman experiences social problems or does not feel sufficient support, an attempt should be made to offer her support and psychotherapy. If a woman's request for CS is due to previous traumatic labour or insufficient pain relief, help should be provided in the form of a consultation with a psychotherapist or a midwife or an analysis of previous labour and pain relief with an obstetrician (Nama and Wilcock, 2011).

CONCLUSION

Major reasons for CDMR include psychological and socio-cultural factors: an "assured" method and date of delivery, previous traumatic experience with labour and labour pain in multiparas, and emotional and social problems. Useful prevention schemes might include a multidisciplinary team, psychotherapeutic assistance started as early as possible, preferably during pregnancy, less industrialised pregnancy and labour, especially for women who have had a traumatic childbirth or insufficient pain relief experience, rediscovery of women's basic needs, physicians' awareness of the psychological aspects of labour pain, and building a patient-obstetrician relationship that is based on mutual cooperation and the use of support psychology. An open discussion on CDMR might bring new insight and inspiration, particularly in the area of social ethics.

In: The Psychological Context of Labour Pain   ISBN: 978-1-63483-825-2
Editors: J. Raudenská and A. Javůrková © 2016 Nova Science Publishers, Inc.

Chapter 6

FEAR OF CHILDBIRTH[*]

*Edita Adamčíková, Iva Korábová,
and Lenka Lacinová*

ABSTRACT

This chapter focuses on the fear of childbirth. Based on a summary of results and findings of previous studies, it discusses its prevalence, aetiology and consequences with a focus on complications that the fear of childbirth can cause during the prenatal, perinatal and postnatal periods. Special attention is given to the causes of the fear of childbirth, which have been divided into "hard" and psychological factors. This classification, as well as the majority of the presented text, is based on an unpublished master thesis by the first author of this chapter – Edita Adamčíková (maiden name Imrychová). At the end of the chapter the recommendations for practices are outlined.

Keywords: fear of childbirth, pregnancy, attachment anxiety and avoidance, satisfaction in romantic relationship, autonomy

[*]The writing of this chapter was partially supported by Student Project Grant at Masaryk University (MUNI/A/1339/2014).

INTRODUCTION

Due to a very low perinatal morbidity and low mortalities of both mothers and newborns in Western countries, it can appear paradoxical that childbirth and the experience of childbirth is for many women significantly impaired by a fear of childbirth (Otley, 2011). Insecurity and anxiety during pregnancy may stem from the women's feeling that they are in a situation where they are facing something unknown which is beyond their control but at the same time inevitable – the upcoming childbirth (Wijma, Wijma and Zar, 1998). The fear of childbirth can be considered to be one of the most common fears during pregnancy. When women were asked about their worries during pregnancy, the most intense or most commonly mentioned concerns were related to worries about birth (Melender, 2002; Öhman, Grunewald and Waldenström, 2003; Peñacoba-Puente, Monge and Morales, 2011). The aim of this chapter is to briefly introduce the phenomenon of the fear of childbirth occurring in pregnancy,[1] its prevalence, aetiology and its possible consequences.

PREVALENCE OF THE FEAR OF CHILDBIRTH

The prevalence of childbirth fear of different intensity among pregnant women ranged between 20-90% (Haines, Rubertsson and Pallant, 2012; Melender, 2002; Öhman, Grunewald and Waldenström, 2003). The fear of childbirth can be classified as being either mild, moderate or severe. The diagnosis of tocophobia (phobia of childbirth) is established when the fear is so intense that the woman in question dreads childbirth and tries to avoid pregnancy (Hofberg and Brockington, 2000; Sydsjö, Sydsjö, Gunnervik, Bladh and Josefsson, 2012).

Even though it is difficult to accurately determine how many pregnant women in the population experience the fear of childbirth in general (as per the wide range mentioned above), available results indicate that approximately 10 to 20% of pregnant women reported severe fear of childbirth (Adams, Eberhard-Gran and Eskild, 2012; Nieminen, Stephansson and Ryding, 2009; Storksen, Eberhard-Gran, Garthus-Niegel and Eskild, 2012).

---

[1] It has been repeatedly verified that fear of childbirth can be experienced by expectant fathers as well (e.g., Hildingsson, Haines, Johansson, Rubertsson, & Fenwick, 2014).

FEAR OF CHILDBIRTH:
CONSEQUENCES DURING PREGNANCY

Melender (2002) identified four main categories of childbirth fear manifestation, which can be concurrently considered as complications caused by the fear of childbirth. The first category was specified as *stress symptoms,* which, for example, included tachycardia, restlessness and nervousness (Melender, 2002). Similarly Nerum, Halvorsen, Sørlie and Øian (2006) reported difficulties with sleep and physiological expressions of fear among all pregnant women suffering from this fear. The second category is described by Melender (2002) as an *influence on everyday life* (tension, anxious child movement counting, excessive limitation of day to day activities, feelings of paranoia and inability to enjoy pregnancy). The third category was defined as the *wish to avoid current pregnancy and childbirth* (desire to postpone pregnancy, thoughts of abortion and feelings of panic connected with the desire to avoid pregnancy and childbirth).

Finally, Melender (2002) described the last category as the *wish to have a caesarean delivery* (under the influence of childbirth fear). A higher incidence of the desire to have a caesarean delivery among pregnant women who experienced strong fear of childbirth was also reported by other studies (Nieminen, Stephansson and Ryding, 2009; Sydsjö G., Sydsjö, A., Gunnervik, Bladh and Josefsson, 2012). Mothers suffering from the fear of childbirth considered vaginal delivery to be hazardous significantly more often and in general they preferred medical interventions during childbirth (Greer, Lazenbatt and Dunne, 2014).

Preterm Birth and Low Birth Weight

Another complication arising in connection with the fear of childbirth is premature birth and the associated low birth weight of newborns. Fear of childbirth can be accompanied by chronic stress to which the body of pregnant woman reacts through endocrinal and immunological responses, which may contribute to preterm birth or low birth weight. For example, increased levels of stress hormones from the hypothalamus and hypophysis are associated with the initiation of preterm childbirth. Angiohypertonia and hypoxia caused by the activation of the sympathetic and adrenal medulla can decrease the blood flow between the placenta and uterus resulting in fetal growth restriction and finally in low birth weight (Dunkel-Schetter, Gurung, Lobel and Wadhwa, 2001). The relationship between premature birth and psychical stress was supported (Staneva, Bogossian, Pritchard and Wittkowski, 2015) as well as the fact that fear of childbirth increases the chances of preterm childbirth (Rondó, Ferreira, Nogueira, Ribeiro, Lobert and Artes, 2003).

Women who delivered a child with lower than standard birth weight often stated that they were experiencing stress throughout almost the whole pregnancy. Furthermore, a higher level of negative attitudes towards pregnancy was identified among these women, in contrast to the women who delivered a child within the standard birth weight limits (Sable and Wilkinson, 2000). This study evaluated the stress experienced during pregnancy and therefore it is possible that the women who delivered a child with a lower childbirth weight than normal could retrospectively evaluate their pregnancy under the influence of this experience. However, stress influences on birth weight were also reported by Rondó Ferreira, Nogueira, Ribeiro, Lobert and Artes (2003), who measured experienced stress during pregnancy. The authors concluded, similarly to Sable and Wilkinson (2000) that the stress experienced during pregnancy influences the child's birth weight, which is often lower than 2500 grams.[2]

FEAR OF CHILDBIRTH: CONSEQUENCES DURING LABOUR

Increased Labour Duration

The duration of labour seems to increase in women with a fear of childbirth (Laursen, Hedegaard and Johansen, 2008). Adams, Eberhard-Gran and Eskild (2012) determined this extra duration to be 47 minutes, taking into account other variables that could affect it. Based on a different study (Sydsjö, G., Angerbjörn, Palmquist, Bladh, Sydsjö A. and Josefsson, 2013), women with a secondary fear[3] of childbirth were in labour for an extra 40 minutes on average, compared to women with no fear of childbirth from control groups.

---

[2] In these studies the low birth weight was related to the immaturity of the newborns, not with the intrauterine growth retardation, therefore the conclusions are again more related to the risk of preterm birth.

[3] Fear of childbirth which was initiated by a previous traumatic childbirth.

Increased Risk of Caesarean Delivery

The results of many studies revealed an increased risk of emergency caesarean delivery in women suffering from a fear of childbirth during pregnancy, compared to women with no fear of childbirth[4] (Adams, Eberhard-Gran and Eskild, 2012;Sydsjö, G., Angerbjörn, Palmquist, Bladh, Sydsjö, A. and Josefsson., 2013). However, studies contradicting this were also published. For example, Johnson and Slade (2002) did not confirm any connection between fear of childbirth during the third trimester and an emergency caesarean delivery or the mode of delivery in general.

Perception of Labour Pain

Alehagen, Wijma and Wijma (2006) found that fear of childbirth measured during the last stage of pregnancy was positively correlated to the fear experienced by women during labour. It is also possible that there is a relation between the fear experienced before and during labour, and the perception of pain during labour. Women who experienced a fear of childbirth during pregnancy reported their labour pain as more intense, compared to women with no fear of childbirth (Haines, Rubertsson, Pallant and Hildingsson, 2012). Alehagen, Wijma K. and Wijma B. (2001) found a relationship between the fear experienced in the early stage of pregnancy and the application of pain relief medication during labour. However, it also needs to be mentioned that some studies did not confirm the relation between fear of childbirth during pregnancy and the intensity of experienced labour pain (Alehagen, Wijma and Wijma 2006). As reported by Lowe (2002), anxiety can influence the perception of childbirth through psychological as well as physiological mechanisms. It mainly increases the release of catecholamines, which then increase the sensitivity of an organism to pain.

---

[4] It is important to remind the reader that the absence of the fear of childbirth does not mean that women do not suffer from any worries in connection with the upcoming childbirth. It only means that these worries have not reached the critical level for the determination of fear of childbirth. This level might differ, based on the measurement criteria used by the research team.

Evaluation of the Childbirth Experience

Women who suffered from fear of childbirth are more likely to evaluate their childbirth as a negative experience. Haines, Pallant, Fenwick, Gamble, Creedy, Toohill and Hildingsson (2015) analysed the responses of women two months after childbirth and found that women who suffered from fear of childbirth were more likely to evaluate their childbirth as a negative experience, compared to women with no fear of childbirth (similarly Elvander, Cnattingius and Kjerulff, 2013; Haines, Rubertsson, Pallant and Hildingsson, 2012).

Similar results were also reported by Waldenström, Hildingsson and Ryding (2006), who found that women suffering from a fear of childbirth during the second trimester and who did not seek professional help, evaluated childbirth as a negative experience significantly more often, regardless of whether the delivery was physiological or via a caesarean. A negative birth experience can be understood not only as a consequence, but also as a cause of fear of childbirth. According to Størksen, Garthus-Niegel, Vangen and Eberhard-Gran (2013), the relationship between previous negative experiences with childbirth and the fear of childbirth is significantly stronger than the relation between fear of childbirth and an actual presence of a clinically measurable delivery complication during previous childbirth. These results emphasize the importance of the subjective perception of childbirth.

FEAR OF CHILDBIRTH: CONSEQUENCES AFTER BIRTH

Feelings of fear and anxiety experienced by women during pregnancy and childbirth also persist after childbirth. Zar, Wijma K. and Wijma B. (2001) found that women who were experiencing mild, moderate or severe fear during pregnancy were experiencing the same levels of fear of childbirth from two hours to five weeks after childbirth. Alehagen, Wijma, B. and Wijma, K. (2006) also concluded that the fear experienced during pregnancy is related to the fear of childbirth that women described two hours, two days and five weeks after childbirth. It was also reported that secondary fear of childbirth prolongs the interval between a traumatic childbirth and following pregnancy (Sydsjö, Angerbjörn, Palmquist, Bladh, Sydsjö and Josefsson, 2013).

Due to the consequences of fear of childbirth presented above, an increasing number of studies point out the necessity of early recognition of the symptoms of fear of childbirth and its early treatment (Nerum, Halvorsen,

Sørlie and Øian, 2006; Otley, 2011; Waldenström, Hildingsson and Ryding, 2006). From the preventative point of view it would be beneficial if specialists were aware of the aetiology of the fear of childbirth and especially of women's characteristics linked to this fear.

Aetiology of the Fear of Childbirth

The causes of the fear of childbirth during pregnancy can be divided into causes of psychological origin (e.g., negative mood), causes of physiological origin (e.g., pregnant woman being ill), external causes (e.g., negative information, a family member being ill), and secondary causes (e.g., previous infertility, previous negative experience with pregnancy, childbirth, health of the child or child care) (Imrychová, 2013). Another division, which will be discussed later in this chapter, is classifying the factors as either "hard" or psychological. "Hard" factors can be represented, for example, by the woman's childbirth history, age, stage of pregnancy and presence or absence of a romantic relationship. Psychological factors include attachment anxiety, avoidance, relationship satisfaction, etc. A study by Imrychová[5] (2013) (for details see Box 1) focused on examining the relationship between the intensity of the fear of childbirth and both "hard" and psychological variables.

"HARD" FACTORS

Age

One would assume that a more intense fear of childbirth will be more prevalent in younger women, as they are more frequently primiparous. Based on the results of a majority of the reviewed studies, primiparous women suffered from a more intense fear of childbirth (Adams, Eberhard-Gran and Eskild, 2012; Melender, 2002; Rouhe, Salmela-Aro, Halmesmäki and Saisto, 2009). In accordance with this assumption, some studies concluded that the incidence of the fear of childbirth decreases with increasing age (Gao, Liu, Fu and Xie, 2015; Laursen, Hedegaard and Johansen, 2008;Peñacoba-Puente, Monge and Morales, 2011). However, there is also evidence that it can occur

---

[5]This part of the chapter is based on the unpublished master thesis of the first author – Edita Adamčíková (Imrychová).

in exactly the opposite way. Bernazzani, Saucier, David and Borgeat (1997) reported that more intense fear and worries were present among older women and similar results were also presented by Nieminen, Stephansson and Ryding, (2009), who found a higher risk of intense fear of childbirth among older women, compared to women aged 25 – 29 years. Other studies, however, did not confirm any significant relationship between the age of pregnant women and the intensity of their experienced fear of childbirth (Zar, Wijma, K. and Wijma, B., 2001).

Box 1. Brief introduction of Imrychová's (2013) study

> The study focused on the fear that women experience during pregnancy specifically with the fear of childbirth. The data was collected from 245 pregnant Czech women aged 18 – 45 years (mean age = 28,99) via the Wijma Delivery Expectancy/Experience Questionnaire, Experience in Close Relationships – Revised – 18, Relationship Assessment Scale (RAS), Basic Psychological Needs Scales – Autonomy scale. Associations between the intensity of fear of childbirth and birth history (last delivery complicated/without complications), anxiety, avoidance, satisfaction in romantic relationships and the subjective feeling of autonomy were found. Relationships with other variables have not been confirmed.

Childbirth History

As has already been stated, the majority of empirical results are in accordance with the assumption that primiparous women experience a more intense fear of childbirth, when compared to parous women. A higher intensity of fear of childbirth is, in this case, associated with the absence of a previous childbirth experience, therefore with the fear of the unknown (Adams, Eberhard-Gran and Eskild, 2012; Rouhe, Salmela-Aro, Halmesmäki and Saisto, 2009). The results of Imrychová's (2013) study are in contradiction to the above mentioned studies, as she did not confirm any significant difference in the average intensity of fear of childbirth between primiparous and parous women. Some research studies indicated that a severe fear of childbirth is more frequently experienced by parous women (Imrychová, 2013; Nieminen, Stephansson and Ryding, 2009). Saisto, Ylikorkala and Halmesmäki (1999) and Melender (2002) reported that a more frequent incidence of severe fear of childbirth among parous women is caused by their traumatic experience from their previous childbirth. Contrastingly, Imrychová (2013) identified only one participant with a severe fear of childbirth who at the same time perceived her previous childbirth as complicated. However, when all the fear intensity categories were taken into account (not only severe fear), the connection between a previous negative experience with childbirth and the intensity of fear of childbirth was found. Women who perceived their last childbirth as complicated experienced a more intense fear of childbirth. It appears that previously experiencing fear increases the probability of the occurrence of the fear of childbirth (Gao, Liu, Fu and Xie 2015), as well as an emergency caesarean delivery (Nilsson, Lundgren, Karlström and Hildingsson, 2012).

Stage of Pregnancy

Many studies confirmed the connection between the intensity of childbirth fear and the stage of pregnancy (Imrychová, 2013; Nieminen, Stephansson and Ryding, 2009; Spice, Jones, Hadjistavropoulos, Kowalyk and Stewart, 2009). Some results described a continuous increase of childbirth fear with increasing stages of pregnancy (Rouhe, Salmela-Aro, Halmesmäki and Saisto, 2009), however, a study by Öhman, Grunewald and Waldenström (2003) revealed a slightly more complicated trajectory, characterized by a decrease of fear intensity in the second trimester and its recurring increase in the third trimester.

Existence of Romantic Relationship

It was found that those women who lived without a partner experienced a more intense fear of childbirth (Haines, Pallant, Fenwick, Gamble, Creedy, Toohill and Hildingsson, 2015; Melender, 2002). The results of quantitative studies are, however, based on a very low number of women without a partner (N = 14 and 11) and it is therefore possible that they are significantly influenced by their low number of respondents. Imrychová (2013) also reported a low number of women who lived without a partner (N = 6), which is one of the limitations of her research. Significant differences in the average values of the experienced fear of childbirth among pregnant women who lived in romantic relationship and women without a partner were not discovered.

PSYCHOLOGICAL FACTORS

Attachment Anxiety

Attachment, which is closely related to the emotional regulation of individual, is an important factor in experiencing fear and its management. Based on the results of previous studies, it appears that the more anxious a woman is, the stronger the fear of childbirth she experiences (Gao, Liu, Fu and Xie, 2015; Imrychová, 2013; Trillingsgaard, Elklit, Shevlin and Maimburg, 2011). Rholes, Simpson, Campbell, and Grich (2001) found that anxious women more often indicated that their partner was not fulfilling their need for attention and support. Anxious women also reported lower marriage satisfaction during pregnancy and after childbirth than women with a secure attachment (also Alexander, Feeney, Hohaus and Noller, 2001).

Haines, Rubertsson, Pallant and Hildingsson (2012) found that fear of childbirth is related to the feelings and concerns of women who lack or will lack the adequate and necessary support during pregnancy and childbirth. It appears that the perception of insufficient support during pregnancy and the concern of not being offered sufficient support in the future, which could be related to the level of anxiety of a woman, can be one of the components of the fear of childbirth. Not just the perception of a partner's insufficient support, but also the overall dissatisfaction in a relationship can be related to the level of anxiety in pregnant women. Trillingsgaard, Elklit, Shevlin and Maimburg (2011) found that a higher level of anxiety is related to lower satisfaction in romantic relationships and to greater stress experienced by both partners during pregnancy. In light of the fact that these studies indicated a relationship between a dissatisfaction in romantic relationships and the occurrence and intensity of the experienced fear of childbirth (Saisto, Salmela-Aro, Nurmi and Halmesmäki, 2001a; Waldenström, Hildingsson and Ryding, 2006), the level of anxiety can be related to the fear of childbirth which is experienced by pregnant women who are dissatisfied in their romantic relationships. Therefore, Trillingsgaard, Elklit, Shevlin and Maimburg (2011) also focused on the direct connection between the level of anxiety of women and fears during pregnancy. They presumed that if the excessive threat perception during confrontation with a stressful situation is one of the symptoms of a higher anxiety level, a greater occurrence of concerns during pregnancy will be detected among women with a higher level of anxiety. The results did confirm this assumption – a higher level of anxiety was connected to the occurrence and intensity of concerns experienced during pregnancy (also Mikulincer and Florian, 1998).

Attachment Avoidance

With respect to the fact that people with an avoidant attachment style tend to rely on themselves in stressful situations and to keep a sufficient distance from other people, it can be presumed that their sensitivity to stressful situations is lower (Mikulincer and Florian, 1998). Trillingsgaard, Elklit, Shevlin and Maimburg (2011) presumed that if sensitivity to stressful situations decreases with an increasing level of avoidance, the connection with intensity of fear during pregnancy should not exist. It is interesting, that based on their results, the authors concluded that a higher level of avoidance as well as a higher level of anxiety were connected to more intense fear experienced during pregnancy. However, this relation was weaker than in the case of anxiety. Other authors concluded similar results (Mikulincer and Florian, 1998; Imrychová, 2013). Similarly to anxiety, it is possible to conclude that fear of childbirth increases with increasing avoidance.

The presented findings are not in accordance with the presumption that a higher level of avoidance relates to a decreasing sensitivity to stressful situations. Therefore, it is possible to suppose that people with higher levels of anxiety, as well as people with higher levels of avoidance perceive stressful situations similarly, but the mechanisms of coping with such situations and their reactions towards the environment are different, due to the dominant dimension of attachment. This would indicate that pregnant women with a higher level of anxiety and a higher level of avoidance perceive the coming childbirth similarly, and in connection to it they experience fear. However, the way they deal with this fear and react to their partner is different. Despite the fact that the fear of childbirth among pregnant women increased with the increasing level of avoidance, the need for their partner during childbirth was decreasing. It is also possible to consider that childbirth can be a very special stressor for avoidant women (the childbirth is obviously connected with some level of women's dependency on the help of others and with future relationship requirements of the dependent child). In the case of anxiety, no connection between attachment style and the need for partner during childbirth was found (Imrychová, 2013).

Satisfaction in Romantic Relationships

Fear of childbirth can also relate to the quality of the romantic relationship the woman is in. Imrychová (2013) found that the less the woman is satisfied in her romantic relationship, the more intense the fear of childbirth she experiences. Negative feelings connected with childbirth were recorded mainly among those women who perceived only very little or no support from their partner (Saisto, Salmela-Aro, Nurmi and Halmesmäki, 2001b; Waldenström, Hildingsson and Ryding, 2006). Similarly to the anxious attachment style, it can be enunciated that the perception of partner support can be related to the attachment of a pregnant woman. Particularly, a high level of anxiety can express itself in a relationship through a chronic feeling of insufficient attention and support from the partner, which can lead to dissatisfaction in the relationship and to a more intense fear of childbirth during pregnancy (Rholes, Simpson, Campbell and Grich, 2001; Trillingsgaard, Elklit, Shevlin and Maimburg, 2011). Nevertheless, it appears that the intensity of fear of childbirth and the dissatisfaction in a relationship increase depending both on anxiety and avoidance (Imrychová, 2013).

Subjective Feeling of Autonomy

Ryding, Wirfelt, Wängborg, Sjögren and Edman (2007) reported that women with a tendency for interpersonal dependency experience fear of childbirth more intensely. Imrychová (2013) also reported a negative relationship between the intensity of fear of childbirth and the subjective feeling of autonomy. Therefore, women who feel more autonomous experience lower levels of fear of childbirth. The author also investigated the relationship between the subjective feeling of autonomy, fear of childbirth and the levels of anxiety and avoidance in pregnant women. It was found that attachment anxiety and avoidance is negatively connected with subjective autonomy and positively with childbirth fear (Imrychová, 2013).

Need for Partner during Childbirth

It can be presumed that higher anxiety expressed through greater fear of childbirth will lead to a greater need for the partner during childbirth, since anxious individuals tend to intensively draw attention onto themselves, if confronted with stressful situations, in order to gain needed support (Trillingsgaard, Elklit, Shevlin and Maimburg, 2011). Imrychová (2013), however, reported that neither a relationship between the need for the partner during childbirth and the intensity of fear of childbirth, nor a relationship between the need for the partner during childbirth and anxiety was found. Her results did however support the presumption that people with a higher level of avoidance tend to rely only on themselves in stressful situations and to keep sufficient distance from other people. Women would not therefore rely so much on the support and reassurance from their partner during pregnancy (Mikulincer and Florian, 1998). The more avoidant the women were, the smaller the need for the partner during childbirth they felt (Imrychová, 2013).

CONCLUSION

Due to possible complications related to the fear of childbirth, extra care should be taken to recognize the symptoms of fear of childbirth at an early stage, in order for it to be treated very early. It would definitely be beneficial to not only have appropriate screening measures[6] available, but also to provide a good overall level of knowledge about the aetiology of the fear of childbirth among doctors. Furthermore, awareness regarding the treatment of fear of childbirth and its prevention should be highlighted not only among researchers but also among experts in practise. There are indications that childbirth education classes of a good quality can have a positive influence (Kızılırmak and Başer, 2015), as well as a childbirth plan and a guarantee of sufficient social support after childbirth (O'Connell, Leahy-Warren, Khashan and Kenny, 2015), guidance and continuous care during labour (Salomonsson, Wijma and Alehagen, 2010) and plenty of space for individual consultancy provided within the frame of fundamental care of women with fear of childbirth (Fenwick, Toohill, Creedy, Smith and Gamble, 2015). Nevertheless there is also some empirical evidence that consultancy addressed towards women with a fear of childbirth alone can be insufficient (Larsson, Karlström, Rubertsson and Hildingsson, 2015). Further research is needed to find more effective programs for treating women with a fear of childbirth.

---

[6]Beside normally used measuring range WDEQ-Q, the Fear of Birth Scale (FOBS) appears to be a suitable tool (Haines et al., 2015).

CONCLUSION

Labour has a very deep meaning; it is a meaningful physiological, psychosocial and spiritual event. The context of labour and birth, pain, suffering, and stress allows certain women to experience labour as a significant event in their lives even though it is painful and uncomfortable. The body, emotions, mind, behaviour and culture are all interconnected. In order to understand labour pain, we need to understand the relationship between life and death, pain and the birth of new life, fear, hope and joy. The value of motherhood, labour and birth, labour pain and suffering, pain relief or no relief should be topics of discussion among experts and the general public. Doctors and other healthcare professionals should be encouraged to create safe spaces for labour where a woman can feel she is in control, pain is perceived as a natural component of labour and birth, and various pharmacological, non-pharmacological and psychological methods of coping with pain are at hand.

ABBREVIATIONS

ASPO	American Society for Psychoprophylaxis in Obstetrics
IPP	Index Present Pain
SF-MPQ	Short form of the McGill Pain Questionnaire
MPQ	McGill Pain Questionnaire
VAS	Visual analogue scale
PBIS	Present Behavioural Intensity Scale
TENS	Transcutaneous electrical nerve stimulation
CS	Caesarean section
PTSD	Post-traumatic stress disorder
CBT	Cognitive Behavioural Therapy
CS	Caesarean section
CSs	Caesarean sections
WHO	World Health Organization
CDMR	Caesarean deliveries on maternal request
USA	United States of America
PTSD	Post-traumatic stress disorder

REFERENCES

Adams, S. S., Eberhard-Gran, M., & Eskild, A. (2012). Fear of childbirth and duration of labour: a study of 2206 women with intended vaginal delivery. *BJOG: An International Journal of Obstetrics and Gynaecology*, 119(10), 1238–1246.

Ajzen, I. (1991). The theory of planned behavior. Organizational Behavior and Human. *Decision Processes*, 50,179 −211.

Ajzen, I., & Fishbein, M. *Understanding attitudes and predicting social behavior.* Englewood Cliffs, NJ: Prentice-Hall, 1980.

Alehagen, S., Wijma, K., & Wijma, B. (2001). Fear during labor. *Acta Obstetriciaet Gynecologica Scandinavica*, 80(4), 315–320.

Alehagen, S., Wijma, K., & Wijma, B. (2006). Fear of childbirth before, during, and after childbirth. *Acta Obstetriciaet Gynecologica Scandinavica*, 85(1), 56–62.

Alexander, R., Feeney, J., Hohaus, L., & Noller, P. (2001). Attachment style and coping resources as predictors of coping strategies in the transition to parenthood. *Personal Relationships*, 8(2), 137–152.

Al-Mufti, R., McCarthy, A., & Fisk, N. M. (1996). Obstetricians´ personal choices and modesof delivery. *Lancet,* 347, 544.

Antonovsky, A. *Health, Stress and Coping.* San Francisco: Jossey-Bass Publisher, 1979.

Andersson, L., Sundström-Poromaa, I., & Bixo, M., et al. (2003). Point prevalence of psychiatric disorders during the second trimester of pregnancy: a population based study. *Am J Obstet Gynecol,* 189, 148–54.

Aslam, M. F., Gilmour, K., & Fawdry, R. D. (2003). Who wants a caesarean section? A study of women´spersonal experineces of vaginal and caesarean delivery. *Journal of Obstetrics and Gynaecology,* 23 (4), 364-366.

Ayers, S., Eagle, A., & Waring, H. (2006). The effects of childbirth-related post-traumatic stress disorder on women and their relationships: a qualitative study. *Psychol Health Med,* 11, 389-98.

Baker, A., Ferguson, S. A., Roach, G. D., & Dawson, D. (2001). Perceptions of labour pain by mothers and their attending midwives. *Journal of Advanced Nursing,* 35(2), 171-179.

Bandura, A. (1997). *Self-efficacy: The exercise of control.* New York, NY: Freeman.

Bandura, A. (1977). Self-efficacy: Toward a unifying theory of behavioural change. *Psychological Review,* 84, 191−215.

Baron, R. S., Logan, H., & Hoppe, S. (1993). Emotional and sensory focus as mediators of dental pain among patients differing in desired and perceived control. *Health Psychology,* 12, 381−389.

Barley, K., Aylin, P., Bottle, A., & Jarman, B. (2004)."Social class and elective Caesareans in the English NHS." *BMJ,* 328 (7453), 1399.

Beauchamp, T. L., & Childress, J. (2001). *Principles of Biomedical Ethics.* Oxford: Oxford University Press.

Beck, N. C., & Hall, D. (1978). Natural Childbirth. A review and analysis. *Obstet Gynec,* 52, 371-379.

Bernat, S. H., Wooldridge, P. J., Marecki, M., & Snell, L. (1992). Biofeedback-assisted relaxation to reduce stress in labor. *J Obstet Gynecol Neonatal Nurs,* 21(4), 295-303.

Bing, E. D. (1994). *Six Practical Lessons for an Easier Childbirth.* New York: Bantam Book.

Bonica, J. J. (1990). *The pain of childbirth.* In Bonica, J. J. (Ed.), *The management of pain* (1313-1343). Malvern, PA: Lea and Febiger.

Bonnel, A. M., & Boureau, F. (1985). Labor pain assessment: validity of a behavioural index. *Pain,* 22(1), 81-90.

Bowlby, J. (1969). *Attachtment. Attachtment and loss.* Harmondsworth: Peguin Books.

Brown, S. T., Campbell, D., & Kurtz, A. (1989). Characteristics of labor pain at two stages of cervical dilation. *Pain,* 38(3), 289-95.

Broome, A. K. (1989). *Health psychology.* London: Chapman and Hall.

Bussche, E., Crombez, G., Eccleston, C., & Sullivan, M. (2007). Why women prefer epidural analgesia during childbirth: The role of beliefs about epidural analgesia and pain catastrophizing. *European Journal of Pain,* 11(3), 275−282.

Büssing, A., Ostermann, T., Neugebauer, E. A. M., Heusser, P. (2010). Adaptive coping strategies in patients with chronic pain conditions and their interpretation of disease. *BMC Public Health*, 10, 507.

Bernazzani, O., Saucier, J. F., David, H., & Borgeat, F. (1997). Psychosocial factors related to emotional disturbances during pregnancy. *Journal of Psychosomatic Research*, *42*(4), 391–402.

Brennan, K. A., Clark, C. L., & Shaver, P., R. (1998). Self-reported measurement of adult attachment: an integrative overview. In Simpson, J. A., & Rholes, S., R. (ed.), *Attachment Theory and Close Relationships* (46–77). London: The Guilford Press.

Burian, J. (1995). Helping survivors of sexual abuse through labor. *The American Journal of Maternal Child Nursing,* 20 (5): 252-256.

Carr, N. (2004). Webwatch. *British Journal of Midwifery*, 12, 514.

Chapman, C. R., & Gavrin, J. (1993). Suffering and its relationship to pain. *J Palliat Care*, 9, 5-13.

Chez, R. A., & Jonas, W. B. (1997). The challenge of complementary and alternative medicine. *Am J Obstet Gynecol,* 177(5), 1156-1161.

Christiaens, W., & Bracke, S. (2007). Assessment of social psychological determinants of satisfaction with childbirth in a cross-national perspective. *BMC Pregnancy and Childbirth*, 26(7), 1-12.

Christiaens, W., Verhaeghe, M., & Bracke, P. (2010). Pain acceptance and personal control in pain relief in two maternity care cross-national comparison of Belgium and the Netherlands. *BMC Health Serv Res*, 10, 268.

Copstick, S., Hayes, R. W., Taylor, K. E., & Morris, N. F. (1985). A test of a common assumption regarding the use of antenatal training during labor. *Journal of Psychosomatic Research*, 29(2), 215-218.

Devendra, K., & Arulkumaran, S. (2003). Should doctors perform elective caesarean sections on request. *Ann Acad Med Singapore,* 32, 577–581; quiz 82.

Dick-Read, G. (1933). *Natural Childbirth.* London: Heineman.

Dick-Read, G. (1944). *Childbirth without fear: The principles and practices of natural childbirth.* New York: Harper and Brothers.

Dick-Read, G. (1959). *Childbirth without fear: The principles and practices of natural childbirth.* New York: Harper and Row.

Dick-Read, G. (1969). *Childbirth without Fear: The Principles and Practice of Childbirth.* New York: Macmillan.

Dick-Read, G., & Wessel, H. (1994). *Childbirth Without Fear: The Original Approach to Natural Childbirth.* New York: Harpercollins.

Dickson, M. J., & Willett, M. (1999). Midwives would prefer a vaginal delivery. *British Medical Journal,* 319, 1008.

Donald, I. & Cooper, S. R. (2001). A Facet Approach to Extending the Normative Component of the Theory of Reasoned Action. *British Journal of Social Psychology,* 40, 599-621.

D'Souza, R., & Arulkumaran, C. (2013). To ´C´ or not to ´C´. Caesarean delivery upon maternal request: a review of facts, figures and guidelines. *Journal of Perinatal Medicine,* 41 (1), 5-15.

Dunkel-Schetter, C. D., Gurung, R. A., Lobel, M., & Wadhwa, P. D. (2001). Stress processes in pregnancy and birth: Psychological, biological, and sociocultural influences. In Baum, A., Revenson, T., & Singer, J. (eds.), *Handbook of health psychology* (495–518). Hillsdale New Jersey: Lawrence Erlbaum.

Easter, A. (2015). Caesarean section should be available on request. Against: Women need accessible evidence-based information on caesarean section. *BJOG,* 2, 359.

Edworthy, Z., Chasey, R., & Williams, H. (2008). The role of schema and appraisals in the development of post-traumatic stress symptoms following birth. *Journal of Reproductive and Infant Psychology,* 26(2), 123–138.

Elvander, C., Cnattingius, S., & Kjerulff, K. H. (2013). Birth Experience in Women with Low, Intermediate or High Levels of Fear: Findings from the First Baby Study. *Birth,* 40(4), 289–296.

Escott, D., Spiby, H., Slade, P., & Fraser, R. B. (2004). The range of coping strategies women use to manage pain and anxiety prior to and during first experience of labor. *Midwifery,* 20,144−156.

Escott, D., Slade, P., Spiby, H., & Fraser, R. B. (2005). Preliminary evaluation of a coping strategy enhancement method of preparation for labor. *Midwifery,* 21, 278−291.

Escott, D., Slade, P., Spiby, H. (2009). Preparation for pain management during childbirth: The psychological aspects of coping strategy development in antenatal education. *Clinical Psychology Review,* 29, 617-622.

Fanning, R. A., Campion, D. P., & Collins, C. B. et al. (2008). A comparison of the inhibitory effects of bupivacaine and levobupivacaine on isolated human pregnant myometrium contractility. *AnesthAnalg,* 107(4), 1303-7.

Fenwick, J., Toohill, J., Creedy, D. K., Smith, J., & Gamble, J. (2015). Sources, responses and moderators of childbirth fear in Australian women: A qualitative investigation. *Midwifery,* 31(1), 239–246.

Fernandez, E., & Turk, D. C. (1989). The utility of cognitive coping strategies for altering pain perception: A meta-analysis. *Pain, 38*, 123−135.

Fillingim, R. B. (2005). *Concise encyclopedia of pain psychology.* New York, London, Oxford: The Haworth Press.

Finger, C. (2003). "Caesarean section rates skyrocket in Brazil." *Lancet, 362* (9384), 628.

Finsen, V., Storeheier, A. H., & Aasland, O. G. (2008). Caesarean section: Norwegian women do as obstetricians do – not as obstetricians say. *Birth,* 35(2), 117-120.

Gee, H. (2015). Caesarean section should be available on request. For: The mother´s autonomy should be paramount. *BJOG,* 2, 359.

Geissbuehler, V., & Eberhard, J. (2002). Fear of childbirth during pregnancy: a study of more than 8000 pregnant women. *J Psychosom Obstet Gynaecol,* 23(4), 229-235.

Gentz, B. A. (2001). Alternative therapies for the management of pain in labor and delivery. *Clin Obstet Gynecol,* 44(4), 704-732.

Graham, W. J., Hundley, V., McCheyne, A. L., Hall, M. H., Gurney, E., & Milne, J. (1999). An investigation of women's involvement in the decision to deliver by caesarean section. *Br J Obstet Gynaecol,* 106, 213-220.

Greer, J., Lazenbatt, A., & Dunne, L. (2014). Fear of childbirth and ways of coping for pregnant women and their partners during the birthing process: a salutogenic analysis. *Evidence Based Midwifery, 12*(3), 1−12.

Gao, L., Liu, X. J., Fu, B. L., & Xie, W. (2015). Predictors of childbirth fear among pregnant Chinese women: A cross-sectional questionnaire survey. *Midwifery, 31*(9), 865–870.

Haines, H. M., Rubertsson, C., Pallant, J. F., & Hildingsson, I. (2012). The influence of women's fear, attitudes and beliefs of childbirth on the mode and experience of birth. *BMC Pregnancy and Childbirth,* 12(1), 55.

Haines, H. M., Pallant, J. F., Fenwick, J., Gamble, J., Creedy, D. K., Toohill, J., & Hildingsson, I. (2015). Identifying women who are afraid of giving birth: A comparison of the fear of birth scale with the WDEQ-A in a large Australian cohort. *Sexual & Reproductive Healthcare.* In press.

Hall, M. H., & Bewley, S. (1999). Maternal mortality and mode of delivery. *Lancet,* 354(9180), 776.

Harrison, A. (1991). Childbirth in Kuwait: the experiences of three groups of Arab mothers. *J Pain Symptom Manager,* 6(8), 466-475.

Henry, A., & Nand, S. (2004). Women's antenatal knowledge and plans regarding intrapartum pain management at the Royal Hospital for Women.

Australian and New Zealand Journal of Obstetrics and Gynaecology, 44, 314–317.

Hildingsson, I., RÍdestad, I., Rubertsson, C., & Waldenström, U. (2002). Few women wish to be delivered by caesarean section. *BJOG,* 109(6), 618–23.

Hildingsson, I., Haines, H., Johansson, M., Rubertsson, C., & Fenwick, J. (2014). Childbirth fear in Swedish fathers is associated with parental stress as well as poor physical and mental health. *Midwifery*, 30(2), 248–254.

Hipwell, A. E., Goossens, F. A., Melhuish, E. C., & Kumar, R. (2000). Severe maternal psychopathology and infant-mother attachment. *Dev Psychopathol*, 12, 157-175.

Hodnett, E. D. (2002). Pain and women's satisfaction with the experience of childbirth: a systematic review. *Am J Obstet Gynecol,* 186 (suppl 5),160-172.

Hofberg, K., & Brockington, I. F. (2000). Tokophobia: an unreasoning dread of childbirth. *The British Journal of Psychiatry*, 176(1), 83–85.

Howard, S. (2003). Imagining the Pain and Peril of Seventeenth century Childbirth: Travail and Deliverance in the Making of an Early Modern World. *Social History of Medicine*; 16(3), 367-382.

Imrychová, E. (2013). *Fear of childbirth: relations and predictors.* Unpublished Master Thesis. Brno: Masarykova univerzita, Fakulta sociálních studií. Available from http://is.muni.cz/th/273090/fss_m_b2/ Edita_Imrychová__273090__Diplomova_prace.pdf.

Janssen, S. A., & Arntz, A. (2001). Real-life stress and opioid-mediated analgesia in novice parachute jumpers. *Journal of Psychophysiology*, 15(3), 106-113.

Johnson, R., & Slade, P. (2002). Does fear of childbirth during pregnancy predict emergency caesarean section? *BJOG: An International Journal of Obstetrics & Gynaecology*, 109(11), 1213–1221.

Jones, L., Othman, M., & Dowswell, T., et al. (2012). Pain management for women in labour: an overview of systematic reviews. *Cochrane Database Syst Rev,* 3: CD009234.

Karmel, M. (1959). *Thank you, Dr. Lamaze, a mother's experiences in painless childbirth.* Philadelphia: Lippincott.

Kennare, R. (2003). Why is the caesarean rate rising? *Midwifery Digest,* 13(4), 503-508.

Kennedy, H. P., Grant, J., Walton, C., Shaw-Battista, J., & Sandall, J. (2010). Normalizing birth in England: a qualitative study. *J Midwifery Womens Health*, 55(3):262-9.

Kitzinger, S. (1996). *The Complete Book of Pregnancy and Childbirth.* New York: Knopf.

Kohl, A., Rief, W., & Glombiewski, J. A. (2013). Acceptance, Cognitive Restructuring, and Distraction as Coping Strategies for Acute Pain. *Journal of Pain*, 14(3), 305–315.

Koerfer, A., Albus, Ch., & Obliers, R. et al. (2008). Kommunikationsmuster der medizinischen Entscheidungsfindung. In Niemeier, S., & Diekmannshenke, H. (Eds.), *Profession und Kommunikation* (121-156). Frankfurt: Lang.

Kızılırmak, A., & Başer, M. (2015). The effect of education given to primigravida women on fear of childbirth. *Applied Nursing Research.* In press.

Lamaze, F. (1956). *Painless childbirth.* New York: Pocket Books.

Lamaze, F. (1972). *Painless Childbirth the Lamaze method.* New York: Pocket Books.

Larsson, B., Karlström, A., Rubertsson, C., & Hildingsson, I. (2015). The effects of counseling on fear of childbirth. *Acta Obstetricia et Gynecologica Scandinavica*, 94(6), 629–636.

Lauer, J. A., Betrán, A. P., Merialdi, M., Wojdyla, D. (2010). *Determinants of caesarean section rates in developed countries: supply, demand and opportunities for control.* World Health Report, Background paper, 29. Geneva: WHO.

Laursen, M., Hedegaard, M., & Johansen, C. (2008). Fear of childbirth: predictors and temporal changes among nulliparous women in the Danish National Birth Cohort. *BJOG: An International Journal of Obstetrics & Gynaecology*, 115(3), 354–360.

Lazarus, R. S. & Folkman, S. (1984). *Stress, Appraisal and Coping.* New York: Springer.

Leboyer, F. (1975). *Birth without violence.* New York: Knopf.

Lefcourt, H. M. (1991). Locus of Control. In Robinson, J. P., Shaver, P. R., & Wrightsman, L. S. (Eds.), *Measures of Personality and Social Psychological Attitudes* (413-499). San Diego: Academic Press.

Ley, P. (1985). Doctor-patient communication: some quantitative estimates of the role of cognitive factors in non-compliance. *J Hypertens Suppl*, 3(1), 51-5.

Lewis, E., & Harris, S. (2010). *Pain relief in labour.* In Clyburn, P., Collis, R., & Harries, S. (ed.), *Obstetric anaesthesia for developing countries* (37-45). New York: Oxford University Press.

Lowe, N. K. (1996). Pain and discomfort of labor and birth. *J Obstet Gynecol Neonatal Nurs,* 25(1), 82-92.

Lowe, N. K. (2002). The nature of labor pain. *Am J Obstet Gynecol,* 186(5), 16-24.

Lowe, N. K. (2000). Self-efficacy for labor and childbirth fears in nulliparous pregnant women. *Journal of Psychosomatic Obstetrics Gynecology,* 21(6), 219-224.

Lundgren, I., & Dahlberg K. (1998). Women's experience of pain during childbirth. *Midwifery;* 14, 105-10.

Mac Kenzie, I. Z. (1999). Should women who elect to have caesarean sections pay for them? *Brit Med J,* 318, 1070.

Mairs, D. (1995). Hypnosis and Pain in Childbirth. *Contemp Hypnosis,* 12(2), 111–118.

Martin, J. A., Hamilton, B. E., Ventura, S. J., Osterman, M. J., Wilson, E. C., & Mathews, T. J. (2012). Births: final data for 2010. *Natl Vital Stat Rep,* 61(1), 22-31.

McCaffery, M., & Pasero, C. (1999). *Pain clinical manual.* St. Louis: Mosby.

McDonald, J. S., & Noback C. R. (2003). Obstetric pain. In Melzack, R., & Wall, P. D. (Ed.), *Handbook of Pain Management. A Clinical Companion to Textbook of Pain* (147 -161). London, Philadelphia: Churchill Livingstone, Elsevier Limited.

Melender, H. L. (2002). Experiences of Fears Associated with Pregnancy and Childbirth: A Study of 329 Pregnant Women. *Birth,* 29(2), 101–111.

Melzack, R. (1984). The myth of painless childbirth (the John J. Bonica lecture). *Pain,* 19(4), 321-337.

Melzack, R. (1987). The short-form McGill Pain Questionnaire. *Pain,* 30 (2), 191–197.

Melzack, R., Taenzer, P., Feldman, P., & Kinch, R. A. (1981). Labour is still painful after prepared childbirth training. *Can Med Assoc J,* 125, 357-63.

Melzack, R., & Schaffelberg, D. (1987). Low-back pain during labor. *Am J Obstet Gynecol,* 156(4), 901-905.

Melzack, R., & Katz, J. (1999). *Pain measurement in persons in pain.* In Wall, P. D., & Melzack, R., (ed.), *Textbook of pain* (337-351). Edinburgh: Churchill Livingstone.

Michaels, P. A. (2012). Pain and Blame: Psychological Approaches to Obstetric Pain, 1950-1980. In Cohen, E., Toker, L., Consonni, M., & Dror, O. (Eds.), *Knowledge and Pain* (231-255). Amsterdam/New York: Rodopi.

Miller, P. M., Fagley, N. S., & Casella, N. E. (2009). Effects of problem frame and gender on principals' decision making. *Social Psychology of Education*, 12(3), 397-413.

Mikulincer, M., & Florian, V. (1998). The relationship between adult attachment styles and emotional and cognitive reactions to stressful events. In Simpson, J. A. & Rholes, W. S. (Ed.), *Attachment theory and close relationships* (143–165). New York, NY, US: Guilford Press.

National Collaborating Centre for Women's and Children's Health. Caesarean Section. Clinical Guideline. London: RCOG Press; 2004 [www.gserve. nice.org.uk/nicemedia/pdf/CG013fullguideline.pdf].

NIH State-of-the-Science Conference Statement on caesarean delivery on maternal request. NIH Consens State Sci Statements 2006; 23:1–29.

Nama, V., & Wilcock, F. (2011). Caesarean section on maternal request: is justification necessary? *The Obstetrician & Gynaecologist*, 13, 263–269.

Nerum, H., Halvorsen, L., Sorlie, T., & Oian, P. (2006). Maternal request for Caesarean Section due to Fear of Birth: Can It Be Changed Through Crisis-Orientated Counselling? *Birth*, 33(3), 221–228.

Nieminen, K., Stephansson, O., & Ryding, E. L. (2009). Women's fear of childbirth and preference for cesarean section – a cross-sectional study at various stages of pregnancy in Sweden. *Acta Obstetricia et Gynecologica Scandinavica*, 88(7), 807–813.

Nilsson, C., Lundgren, I., Karlström, A., & Hildingsson, I. (2012). Self reported fear of childbirth and its association with women's birth experience and mode of delivery: A longitudinal population-based study. *Women and Birth*, 25(3), 114–121.

Niven, C. A., & Gijsbers, K. (1984). A study of labour pain using the McGill Pain Questionnaire. *Soc Sci Med*, 19(12), 1347-1351.

Niven, C. A., & Gijsbers, K. (1996). Coping with labor pain. *J Pain Symptom Management*, 11(2), 116-125.

Niven, C. A., & Murphy-Black, T. (2000). Memory for Labor Pain: A Review of the Literature. *Birth*, 27(4), 244–253.

O'Connell, M., Leahy-Warren, P., Khashan, A. S., & Kenny, L. C. (2015). Tocophobia – the new hysteria? *Obstetrics, Gynaecology and Reproductive Medicine*, 25(6), 175–177.

Odent, M. (2004). *The caesarean*. London: Free Associations Books.

Odent, M. (2007). *Birth reborn. What childbirth should be*. New York: Souvenir Press.

Öhman, S. G., Grunewald, C., & Waldenström, U. (2003). Women's worries during pregnancy: testing the Cambridge Worry Scale on 200 Swedish women. *Scandinavian Journal of Caring Sciences*, 17(2), 148–152.

Otley, H. (2011). Fear of childbirth: Understanding the causes, impact and treatment. *British Journal of Midwifery*, *19*(4), 215–220.

Pasero, C., & McCaffery, M. (2011). *Pain: Assessment and pharmacologic management*. Missouri St Louis: Mosby Elsevier.

Pesce, G. (1987). Measurement of reported pain of childbirth: a comparison between Australian and Italian subjects. *Pain,* 31(1), 87-92.

Peñacoba-Puente, C., Monge, F. J. C., & Morales, D. M. (2011). Pregnancy worries: a longitudinal study of Spanish women. *Acta Obstetricia et Gynecologica Scandinavica*, 90(9), 1030–1035.

Potter, J. E., Berquó, E., Perpétuo, I. H., Leal, O. F., Hopkins, K., & Souza, M. R., et al. (2001). Unwanted caesarean sections among public and private patients in Brazil: prospective study. *BMJ*, 323:1155–8.

Potter, J. E., & Hopkins, K. (2002). Consumer demand for caesarean sections in Brazil. Demand should be assessed rather than inferred. *BMJ*, 325, 335.

Price, D. D. (2002). Central Neural Mechanisms that Interrelate Sensory and Affective Dimensions of Pain. *Molecular Interventions*, 2, 392-403.

Quadros, L. (2000). Brazilian obstetricians are pressured to perform caesarean sections. *Brit Med J,* 320, 1073.

Raudenska, J., Javurkova, A., & Kozak, J. (2013). Fear of pain and movement in a patient with musculoskeletal chronic pain. *Neuronedocrinol Lett*, 34, (6), 101-104.

Raudenska, J., Amlerova, J., & Javurkova, A. (2014). Cognitive behavioral therapy in pain management of adult chronic nonmalignant pain patients. In Myers, B. (ed.), *Cognitive Behavioral Therapy: New Research* (79-100). New York: Nova Science Publisher.

Ramirez-Maestre, C., Esteve, R., & Lopez, A. E. (2008). Cognitive appraisal and coping in chronic pain patients. *Eur J Pain*, 12, 749-756.

Rholes, W. S., Simpson, J. A., Campbell, L., & Grich, J. (2001). Adult attachment and the transition to parenthood. *Journal of Personality and Social Psychology*, *81*(3), 421–435.

Rokke, P. D., & Al'Absi, M. (1992). Matching pain coping strategies to the individual. A prospective validation of the cognitive coping strategy inventory. *Journal of Behavioral Medicine*, 15, 611−625.

Rokke, P. D., & Lall, R. (1992). The role of choice in enhancing tolerance to acute pain. *Cognitive Therapy and Research*, 16, 53−65.

Rondó, P. H. C., Ferreira, R. F., Nogueira, F., Ribeiro, M. C. N., Lobert, H., & Artes, R. (2003). Maternal psychological stress and distress as predictors of low birth weight, prematurity and intrauterine growth retardation. *European Journal of Clinical Nutrition*, 57(2), 266–272.

Rossi, A. C., & D'Addario, V. (2008). Maternal morbidity following a trial of labour after caesarean section vs elective repeat caesarean delivery: a systematic review with metaanalysis. *Am J Obstet Gynecol*, Sept, 224–231.

Rothbaum, R., Weiss, J. R., & Snyder, S. S. (1982). Changing the world and changing the self: a two-process model of perceived control. *J Pers & Soc Psych*, 42, 5-37.

Rotter, J. (1966). Generalized expectancies for internal versus external control of reinforcements. *Psychological Monographs*, 80, 609.

Rouhe, H., Salmela-Aro, K., Halmesmäki, E. & Saisto, T. (2009). *Fear of childbirth according to parity, gestational age, and obstetric history*. *BJOG*, 116(1), 67-73.

Ruble, D. N., Brooks-Gunn, J., Fleming, A. S., Fitzmaurice, G., Stangor, C., & Deutsch, F. (1990). Transition to motherhood and the self: measurement, stability, and change. *J Pers Soc Psychol*, 58, 450-463.

Ruppen, W., Derry, S., McQuay, H., & Moore, R. A. (2006). Incidence of epidural hematoma, infection and neurologic injury in obstetric patients with epidural analgesia/anesthesia. *Anestesiology*, 105 (2), 394-399.

Ryding, E. L. (1993). Investigation of 33 women who demanded a cesarean section for personal reasons. *Acta Obstet Gynecol Scand*, 72, 280–5.

Ryding, E. L., Wijma, B., & Wijma, K. (1997). Posttraumatic stress reactions after emergency cesarean section. *Acta Obstet Gynecol Scand,* 76, 856-861.

Ryding, E. L., Wirfelt, E., Wängborg, I.-B., Sjögren, B., & Edman, G. (2007). Personality and fear of childbirth. *Acta Obstetricia Et Gynecologica Scandinavica*, 86(7), 814–820.

Sable, M. R., & Wilkinson, D. S. (2000). Impact of perceived stress, major life events and pregnancy attitudes on low birth weight. *Family Planning Perspectives*, 32(6), 288–294.

Saisto, T., Ylikorkala, O., & Halmesmäki, E. (1999). Factors associated with fear of delivery in second pregnancies. *Obstetrics and Gynecology*, 94(5 Pt 1), 679–682.

Saisto, T., Salmela-Aro, K., Nurmi, J. E., & Halmesmäki, E. (2001a). Psychosocial characteristics of women and their partners fearing vaginal childbirth. *BJOG: An International Journal of Obstetrics and Gynaecology*, 108(5), 492–498.

Saisto, T., Salmela-Aro, K., Nurmi, J. E., & Halmesmäki, E. (2001b). Psychosocial predictors of disappointment with delivery and puerperal depression. A longitudinal study. *Acta Obstet Gynecol Scand,80*(1), 39-45.

Saisto, T., Kaaja, R., Ylikorkala, O., & Halmesmäki, E. (2001). Reduced pain tolerance during and after pregnancy in women suffering from fear of labor. *Pain,* 93(2),123-127.

Saisto, T., & Halmesmäki, E. (2003). Fear of childbirth: a neglected dilemma. *Acta Obstet Gynecol Scand*, 82(3), 201-208.

Salomonsson, B., Wijma, K., & Alehagen, S. (2010). Swedish midwives' perceptions of fear of childbirth. *Midwifery*, 26(3), 327–337.

Sawyer, A., & Ayers, S. (2009). Post-traumatic growth in women after childbirth. *Psychology and Health,* 24(4), 457–471.

Seeman, M. Alienation studies. *Annu Rev Sociol*, 1975, 1, 91-123.

Seeman, M. Alienation and Anomie. (1991). In Robinson, J. P., Shaver, P. R., & Wrightsman, L. S. (Eds), *Measures of Personality and Social Psychological Attitudes* (291-372). San Diego: Academic Press.

Seligman, M. (1975). *Helplessness: On depression, development, and death.* San Francisco: Freeman.

Senden, I. P., Wetering, M. D., Eskes, T. K., Biewrkens, P. B., Laube, D. W. & Pitkin, R. M. (1988). Labor pain: a comparison of parturients in a Dutch and an American teaching hospital. *ObstetGynecol,* 71(4), 541-544.

Sheiner, E. K., Sheiner, E., Shoham-Vardi, I., Mazor, M., & Katz, M. (1999). Ethnic differences influence care giver's estimates of pain during labour. *Pain,* 81(3), 299-305.

Sheiner, E., Sheiner, E. K., Hershkovitz, R., Mazor, M., Katz, M., & Shoham-Vardi, I. (2000). Overestimation and underestimation of labor pain. *Eur J Obstet Gynecol Reprod Biol,* 91(1), 37-40.

Schenker, J. G., & Cain, J. M. (1999). FIGO Committee Report. FIGO Committee for the Ethical Aspects of Human Reproduction and Women's Health. International Federation of Gynaecology and Obstetrics. *Int J Gynaecol Obstet*, 64, 317–22.

Schultz, R., Heckhausen, J. & O'Brian, AT. Control and the disablement process in the elderly. *J Soc Beh and Pers,* 1994, 9, 139-152.

Simkin, P. & O'Hara, M. (2002). Nonpharmacologic relief of pain during labor: systematic review of five Metod. *Am J Obstet Gynaecol,* 186, Suppl 5, 131-159.

Sjögren, B., & Thomassen, P. (1997). Obstetric outcome in 100 women with severe anxiety over childbirth. *Acta Obstet Gynecol Scand*, 76, 948-952.

Slade, P., Escott, D., Spiby, H., Henderson, B., & Fraser, R. B. (2000). Antenatal predictors and use of coping strategies in labor. *Psychology and Health*, 15, 555−569.

Söderquist, J., Wijma, B., & Thorbert, G., et al. (2009). Risk factors in pregnancy for posttraumatic stress and depression after childbirth. *BJOG*, 116, 672–80.

Spiby, H., Slade, P., Escott, D., Henderson, B., & Fraser, R. B. (2003). Selected coping strategies in labor: An investigation of women's experiences. *Birth: Issues in Perinatal Care*, 30, 189−194.

Spice, K., Jones, S. L., Hadjistavropoulos, H. D., Kowalyk, K., & Stewart, S. H. (2009). Prenatal fear of childbirth and anxiety sensitivity. *Journal of Psychosomatic Obstetrics and Gynaecology*, 30(3), 168–174.

Staneva, A., Bogossian, F., Pritchard, M., & Wittkowski, A. (2015). The effects of maternal depression, anxiety, and perceived stress during pregnancy on preterm birth: A systematic review. *Women and Birth*. In press.

Stevens, B., Watt-Watson, J., & Gibbins, S. (2003). Psychological therapies. In Rowbotham, D. J., & Macintyre, P. E. (Eds.), *Acute pain* (36-39). London: Arnold.

Storksen, H. T., Eberhard-Gran, M., Garthus-Niegel, S., & Eskild, A. (2012). Fear of childbirth; the relation to anxiety and depression. *ActaObstetricia Et Gynecologica Scandinavica*, 91(2), 237–242.

Størksen, H. T., Garthus-Niegel, S., Vangen, S., & Eberhard-Gran, M. (2013). The impact of previous birth experiences on maternal fear of childbirth. *Acta Obstetricia et Gynecologica Scandinavica*, 92(3), 318–324.

Sullivan, M. J., Rodgers, W. M., & Kirsch, I. (2001). Catastrophizing, depression and expectancies for pain and emotional distress. *Pain*, 91, 147−154.

Svensson, J., Barclay, L., & Cooke, M. (2008). Effective Antenatal Education: Strategies Recommended by Expectant and New Parents. *J Perinat Educ*, 17(4), 33–42.

Sydsjö, G., Sydsjö, A., Gunnervik, C., Bladh, M., & Josefsson, A. (2012). Obstetric outcome for women who received individualized treatment for fear of childbirth during pregnancy. *Acta Obstetricia Et Gynecologica Scandinavica*, 91(1), 44–49.

Sydsjö, G., Angerbjörn, L., Palmquist, S., Bladh, M., Sydsjö, A., & Josefsson, A. (2013). Secondary fear of childbirth prolongs the time to subsequent delivery. *Acta Obstetricia Et Gynecologica Scandinavica*, 92(2), 210–214.

Szeverenyi, P., Poka, R., Hetey, M., & Torok, Z. (1998). Contents of childbirth-related fear among couples wishing the partner's presence at delivery. *J Psychosom Obstet Gynaecol*, 19, 38-43.

Taenzer, P. (1983). Post-operative pain: Relationships among measures of pain, mood and narcotic requirements. In Melzack, R. (Ed.), *Pain measurement and assessment* (51-63). New York: Raven.

Thompson, S. C. (1981). A complex answer to a simple question: Will it hurt less if I can control it? *Psychological Bulletin*, 90, 89-101.67.

Thompson, S. C., & Spacapan, S. (1991). Perceptions of control in vulnerable populations. *Journal of Social Issues*, 47, 1-21.

Torloni, M. R., Betrán, A. P., Montilla, P., Scolaro, E., Seuc, A., Mazzoni, A., Althabe, F., Merzagora, F., Donzelli G., P., & Merialdi, M. (2013). Do Italian women prefer cesarean section? Results from a survey on mode of delivery preferences. *BMC Pregnancy and Childbirth*, 13, 78.

Tournaire, M., & Theau-Yonneau A. (2007). Complementary and Alternative Approaches to Pain Relief During Labor. *Evid Based Complement Alternat Med*, 4(4), 409–417.

Tranquilli, A. L., & Garzetti, G. G. (1997). A new ethical and clinical dilemma in obstetric practice: caesarean section "on maternal request." *Am J ObstetGynecol*, 177, 245-246.

Trillingsgaard, T., Elklit, A., Shevlin, M., & Maimburg, R. D. (2011). Adult attachment at the transition to motherhood: predicting worry, health care utility and relationship functioning. *Journal of Reproductive and Infant Psychology*, 29(4), 354–363.

Tsui, M. H., Pang, M. W., Melender, K. L., Xu, L., Lau, T. K., & Lejny, T. N. (2006). Maternal fear associated with pregnancy and childbirth in Hong Kong Chinese women. *Women and Health*, 44(4), 79-92.

Usha Kiran T. S., & Jayawickrama, N. S. (2002). "Who is responsible for the rising Caesarean section rate?" *J Obstet Gynaecol*, 22 (4), 363–5.

Van der Kolk, B. A., & Fisler, R. (1995). Dissociation & the Fragmentary Nature of Traumatic Memories: Overview and Exploratory Study. *Journal of Traumatic Stress*, 8(4), 505-525.

Verdult, R. (2009). Caesarean birth: Psychological aspects in babies. *Journal of Prenatal and Perinatal Psychology and medicine*, 21 (1/2), 29-41.

Vick, S., & Scott, A.(1998). Agency in health care. Examining patient's preferences for attributes of the doctor-patient relationship. *Journal of Health Economics*, 17(5), 587-605.

Vlaeyen, J. W. S., Morley, S., Linton, SJ., Boersma, K., & De Jong, J. (2012). *Pain-Related Fear: Exposure-Based Treatment for Chronic Pain.* Seattle: IASP Press.

Zar, M., Wijma, K., & Wijma, B. (2001). Pre- and Postpartum Fear of Childbirth in Nulliparous and Parous Women. *Scandinavian Journal of Behaviour Therapy*, 30(2), 75–84.

Zhang, J., Liu, Y., Meikle, S., Zheng, J., Sun, W., & Li, Z. (2008). "Caesarean delivery on maternal request in southeast China." *Obstet Gynecol,*111 (5), 1077–82.

Wagner, M. (1994). *Pursuing the birth machine; the search for appropriate birth technology.* Camperdown: ACE Graphics.

Waldenström, U. (2004). Why Do Some Women Change Their Opinion About Childbirth Over Time? *Birth,* 31(2), 102–107.

Waldenström, U., Hildingsson, I., Rubertsson, C., & Rådestad, I. (2004). A Negative Birth Experience: Prevalence and Risk Factors in a National Sample. *Birth,* 31(1), 17–27.

Waldenström, U., Hildingsson, I., & Ryding, E. (2006). Antenatal fear of childbirth and its association with subsequent caesarean section and experience of childbirth. *BJOG: An International Journal of Obstetrics and Gynaecology,* 113(6), 638-646.

Waters, D. C. (1998). *Just take it out.* Mt. Vernon, Ill: Topiary Publishing,.

Weisenberg, M., & Caspi, Z. (1989). Cultural and educational influences on pain of childbirth. *J Pain Symptom Manager,* 4(1), 13-9.

Wewers, M. E., & Lowe, N. K. (1990). A critical review of visual analogue scales in the measurement of clinical phenomena. *Res Nurs Health,* 13 (4), 227-236.

WHO Statement on Caesarean Section Rates. (2015). Geneva: WHO.

World health statistics. (2014). Geneva: WHO.

Wijma, K., Wijma, B., & Zar, M. (1998). Psychometric aspects of the W-DEQ; a new questionnaire for the measurement of fear of childbirth. *Journal of Psychosomatic Obstetrics and Gynaecology*, 19(2), 84–97.

Wiklund, I., Edman, G., & Andolf, E. (2007). Cesarean section on maternal request: reasons for the request, self-estimated health, expectations, experience of birth and signs of depression among first-time mothers. *Acta Obstetricia et Gynecologica Scandinavica,* 86(4), 451–456.

Wiklund, I., Edman, G., Ryding, E. L., & Andolf, E. (2008). Expectation and experiences of childbirth in primiparae with caesarean section. *BJOG*, 115, 324–31.

Wiklund, I., Edman, G., Larsson, C, & Andolf E. (2009). First-time mothers andchanges in personality in relation to mode of delivery. *J AdvNurs*, 65, 1636–44.

Wiklund, I., Andolf, E., Lilja, H., & Hildingsson, I. (2012). Indications for caesarean section on maternal request – Guidelines for counseling and treatment. *Sexual & Reproductive Healthcare,* 3, 99-106.

Winsberg, B., & Greenlick, M. (1967). Pain response in Negro and white obstetrical patients. *J Health Soc Behav,* 8(3), 222-227.

Winterowd, C., Beck, A. T., & Gruener, D. (2003). *Cognitive therapy with chronic pain patients.* New York: Springer Publishing Co.

Wuitchik, M., Hesson, K., & Bakal, D. A. (1990). Perinatal predictors of pain and mistress during labor. *Birth,* 17,186–191.

ABOUT THE AUTHORS

Jaroslava Raudenská, Dr., PhD
Clinical Psychologist and Cognitive Behavioural Therapist
Department of Nursing, 2nd Faculty of Medicine
Charles University and Motol University Hospital
Prague, the Czech Republic
Department of Clinical Psychology, Motol University Hospital
Prague, the Czech Republic
Email: jaroslava.raudenska@fnmotol.cz

Jaroslava completed her psychology studies at the Faculty of Arts of the Charles University in Prague, the Czech Republic. She is a registered clinical psychologist and cognitive behavioural therapist and works as the head of the Department of Clinical Psychology of the Motol University Hospital in Prague. Her speciality is psychological diagnostics and psychotherapy in patients with acute and chronic cancer pain and non-cancer related pain. She gives lectures on medical psychology and the psychology of pain as part of the under-graduate education of medical students, nurses and other practitioners at the 2nd Faculty of Medicine of the Charles University in Prague; she also gives lectures as part of the post-graduate education of medical doctors – algesiologists, palliative medicine specialists, rehabilitative medicine specialists and clinical psychologists at the Institute for postgraduate medical education in Prague.

Alena Javůrková, Dr., PhD
Clinical Psychologist and Cognitive Behavioural Therapist
Department of Nursing, 2nd Faculty of Medicine
Charles University and Motol University Hospital
Prague, the Czech Republic,
Department of Clinical Psychology, KV University Hospital,
Prague, the Czech Republic
Email: alena.javurkova@post.cz

Alena completed her psychology studies at the Faculty of Arts of the Charles University in Prague, the Czech Republic. She is a registered clinical neuropsychologist and cognitive behavioural therapist and works as the head of the Department of Clinical Psychology of the Královské Vinohrady University Hospital in Prague. Her speciality is the neuropsychological testing of cognitive functions. In cooperation with the Motol University Hospital she engages in pre-operative examination of cognitive functions in epileptic patients. In psychotherapy she specialises in coping with chronic disease. She gives lectures on medical psychology (needs in the context of the nursing process and research in nursing) and pedagogical psychology as part of the under-graduate education of medical students and nurses at the 2nd Faculty of Medicine of the Charles University in Prague; she also gives lectures on neuropsychology as part of the post-graduate education of clinical psychologists, medical doctors and physiotherapists.

Jana Amlerová, MD, PhD
Department of Neurology, 2nd Faculty of Medicine
Charles University in Prague and Motol University Hospital
Prague, the Czech Republic

Antonella Paladini, MD, Ass. Professor
Department of Anesthesiology and Pain Medicine
University of L'Aquila, Italy

Edita Adamčíková, MA
Faculty of Social Studies, Masaryk University
Brno, the Czech Republic
Email: edi.adamcikova@gmail.com

Iva Korábová, MA
Institute for Research on Children, Youth and Family
Faculty of Social Studies, Masaryk University
Brno, the Czech Republic

Lenka Lacinová, MA, PhD, Ass. Professor
Institute for Research on Children, Youth and Family,
Faculty of Social Studies, Masaryk University, Brno, the Czech Republic

Reviewed by:

Dr. Ellena Huse
Registered Psychologist and Psychotherapist
University of Education, Freiburg, Germany

Ass. Prof. Dr. Thomas Meuser
Head of Department of Anaesthesiology
Marienkrankenhaus Bergisch Gladbach, Germany

Prof. Giustino Varrassi
President
Paolo Procacci Foundation and President European League
Against Pain (EULAP), Rome, Italy

SUPPORT

This book was supported by the Ministry of Health, Czech Republic - conceptual development of research organization, University Hospital Motol, Prague, Czech Republic 00064203.

INDEX